皮肤病治疗系列

肿瘤治疗的皮肤反应
Dermatologic Reactions to Cancer Therapies

主 编
[意] 加布里埃拉·法布罗奇尼(Gabriella Fabbrocini)
[美] 马里奥·拉库蒂尔(Mario E. Lacouture)
[美] 安东内拉·托斯蒂(Antonella Tosti)

主 译
盛友渔　张　波

主 审
王侠生　陈连军

復旦大學出版社

译审者名单

主　审　王侠生　复旦大学附属华山医院
　　　　　陈连军　复旦大学附属华山医院
主　译　盛友渔　复旦大学附属华山医院
　　　　　张　波　复旦大学附属肿瘤医院
译　者　金尚霖　复旦大学附属华山医院
　　　　　韩中颖　上海市中医医院
　　　　　齐思思　复旦大学附属华山医院
　　　　　胡瑞铭　复旦大学附属华山医院
　　　　　刘孟国　复旦大学附属华山医院
　　　　　周丽娟　复旦大学附属华山医院
　　　　　杨凡萍　复旦大学附属华山医院
　　　　　赵　俊　复旦大学附属华山医院
　　　　　赵　颖　复旦大学附属华山医院
　　　　　缪　盈　复旦大学附属华山医院
　　　　　王轶伦　复旦大学附属华山医院
　　　　　刘　晓　复旦大学附属华山医院
　　　　　陶　璐　复旦大学附属华山医院

主审简介

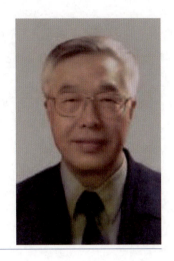

王侠生 教授,博士生导师。

1957年毕业于上海第一医学院医疗系皮肤性病学专业;1981—1984年于美国辛辛那提大学医学中心研修职业性环境性皮肤病及皮肤毒理学。曾任上海医科大学皮肤病学研究所所长,附属华山医院皮肤科主任;兼任亚洲皮肤科协会理事,中华医学会皮肤科学会委员,上海市皮肤科学会主任委员等;《中华皮肤科杂志》副主编,《临床皮肤科杂志》《中国皮肤性病学杂志》《中国麻风皮肤病杂志》等编委。主要研究领域是职业性环境性皮肤病、皮肤毒理及变应性免疫性皮肤病等。在国内外刊物发表论文120余篇。主编皮肤科教材、参考书及工具书共18部,包括《皮肤病学》《职业性及环境性皮肤病》《皮肤科用药及其药理》《杨国亮皮肤病学》《现代皮肤病学》《皮肤科手册》等。先后培养硕士生、博士生21名。获部、市级科技奖8项。1991年被评为校优秀教育工作者;1992年起享受国务院颁发的政府特殊津贴。

主审简介

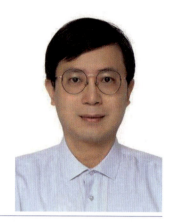

陈连军 复旦大学附属华山医院皮肤科副主任医师,皮肤病理室顾问。

1999年毕业于上海医科大学,获临床医学硕士学位;2006年获复旦大学临床医学博士学位。2006年8月至2007年7月在美国宾西法尼亚大学附属医院学习。现任上海市医学会皮肤科分会病理学组组长,中华医学会病理学分会委员,中华医学会皮肤性病学分会病理学组委员,中国医师协会皮肤科医师分会病理亚专业委员会委员,中国中西医结合学会皮肤性病专业委员会青年委员。从事皮肤科临床和病理工作20余年,擅长特异性皮炎、少见和疑难皮肤病的诊断和治疗,倡导临床、影像学和病理学相结合的皮肤病诊断模式。2013年获中国医师协会皮肤科医师分会优秀中青年医师奖,2014年获上海市住院医师规范化培训优秀带教老师。先后在国内外期刊以第一作者或通信作者发表论文20余篇,参编或参译专著7部,副主译专著1部,参加多项上海市和国家自然科学基金项目,主持上海市卫健委科研项目2项。

主译简介

盛友渔 医学博士,复旦大学附属华山医院皮肤科主治医师。

先后在复旦大学上海医学院获得七年制临床医学硕士和皮肤病学博士学位。上海市医学会皮肤性病学会毛发学组、上海市中医药学会皮肤病分会毛发学组、中国非公医疗皮肤专委会毛发医学与头皮健康管理学组、中国抗衰老医学美容协会头皮与毛发学组成员。主攻重症斑秃、中重度女性型脱发、休止期脱发、慢性活动性EB病毒感染、肿瘤相关皮肤反应等疾病的发病机制和临床治疗研究。担任《中国美容医学》杂志编委,参编专著《现代皮肤病学》。主译《斑秃:临床医师手册》《毛发疾病的诊断与治疗技术》。

主译简介

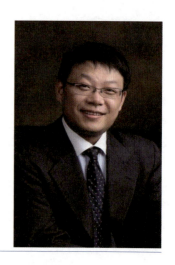

张 波 医学博士,复旦大学附属肿瘤医院胰腺外科主任医师,硕士生导师,复旦大学附属肿瘤医院医务部副主任、浦东院区医疗综合办主任。

先后在复旦大学上海医学院获得七年制临床医学硕士和外科学博士学位。以第一作者或通讯作者发表SCI收录论文10余篇,承担国家自然科学基金面上项目1项,上海市科委和卫健委课题各1项。

Translator's Preface

译 者 序

近十几年来恶性肿瘤的发病率和死亡率呈上升趋势，恶性肿瘤/癌症已成为一个重大的公共卫生问题。2022年2月，国家癌症中心发布了最新一期的全国癌症统计数据，我国癌症发病率仍然呈现上升趋势，每年癌症所致的医疗花费超过2 200亿元。

肿瘤治疗主要包括传统的手术治疗、放疗、化疗、中医中药和近年来发展迅速的靶向治疗、免疫治疗、过继性T细胞治疗和造血干细胞移植等，临床上通常联合应用多种治疗手段以提高疗效。过去几十年里，抗肿瘤疗法研发取得了很多突破性进展。以靶向治疗为例，美国食品药品监督管理局（FDA）已批准了针对30余种靶点的靶向治疗药物，为对传统治疗无效的肿瘤患者带来了新的希望。然而，与此同时，这些新型疗法引起的不良事件也越来越成为临床常见而亟待解决的问题。皮肤不良反应不仅会损害患者的身体功能和生活质量，还会导致药物剂量减少、治疗方案修改甚至抗肿瘤治疗中断，最终对肿瘤患者的预后造成负面甚至危及生命的影响。

本书引自国际知名的泰勒-弗朗西斯出版集团CRC出版社（CRC Press LLC/Taylor & Francis），是一部最新的（原著于2019年3月出版）介绍肿瘤治疗相关皮肤反应诊疗策略的专著。原著主编Gabriella Fabbrocini教授、Mario E. Lacouture教授和Antonella Tosti教授均是该专业领域的权威，3位专家凭借深厚的理论功底和丰富的实践经验，全面、详尽地介绍了每种皮肤不良事件的诊断、评估与治疗，配以丰富的病例照片，将要点、难点整理总结成图表，便于读者在临床工作中借鉴。

我在2021年底病房带组期间阅读到本书原著，当时病房接连收治了好几例恶性肿瘤合并疑难危重皮肤病患者，在遇到临床难题时读到本书有种如获至宝的感受。之后我和组里的同道一致愿意将本书翻译成中文版，希望有助于提升大家对于肿瘤治疗相关皮肤反应的认知和处理水平。衷心感谢参与本书翻译的各位同道所付出的辛勤努力。我荣幸地邀请到复旦大学附属肿瘤医院张波教授和我一起担任本书主译，他是一位胰腺外科专家，在肿瘤治疗术语方面提供了许多专业指导。极其荣幸能够邀请到王侠生教授和陈连军教授担任本书主审，衷心感谢两位教授的悉心指导和支持。我还要感谢复旦大学出版社对我们的信任，以及在编辑和出版事务方面给予的支持和帮助。

正如原著主编Mario E Lacouture教授所说，新疗法的迅速发展带来了有希望的抗肿瘤疗效，但同时也带来了各种新的不良反应。皮肤不良事件是最常见的，可能严重影响患者的生活质量，并且牵涉肿瘤的维持治疗。通过全面、规范的治疗前评估、早期诊断和适当处理，这些皮肤不良事件是可以预防和控制的。皮肤科医生在减少皮肤不良事件的影响方面发挥着关键作用。早期、及时的皮肤科会诊和包括皮肤科医生在内的多学科团队有助于优化肿瘤的治疗。

限于译者的水平，本书错漏缺点在所难免，敬请各位同道和广大读者批评指正。

复旦大学附属华山医院皮肤科　盛友渔
2022 年 9 月

非常高兴，有机会接受盛友渔医生的邀请，参与 Dermatologic Reactions to Cancer Therapies（《肿瘤治疗的皮肤反应》）这一英文原版著作的翻译工作。确实，对于肿瘤治疗中的，尤其是放化疗引起的皮肤反应性疾病的认识，是我们肿瘤专科医生所缺乏或者容易忽略的，从而导致临床处置的延误或者耽搁。

在翻译本书的过程中，我最直接的感受就是，化疗药物所引起的各类皮肤反应性疾病的不同表现形式，对于皮肤科医生来说是有挑战的。不同化疗药物的不同作用机制，所表现出来的不同症状，均需要皮肤科医生给予严格的对症处理；同时也让我们肿瘤专科医生了解到放化疗药物、射线等引起的皮肤反应是可以导致严重并发症的，严重的可能导致肿瘤治疗的延误或者失败，由此带给患者的将是心理和身体的双重打击。通过本书的翻译和介绍，可以让相关肿瘤专业医生和皮肤科医生一起探讨和研究肿瘤治疗过程中皮肤反应的治疗对策和方法，减轻因为化疗药物或者射线引起的皮肤反应，保障肿瘤患者得到充分有效的治疗，从而改善患者的生活质量和生存状态。

希望本书可以给所有从事肿瘤治疗的医生、皮肤科医生等有章可循，有据可查。在翻译过程中，因为译者的水平有限，可能存在词不达意的情况，也请读者给予批评指正，以利于工作的持续改进。

复旦大学附属肿瘤医院　张波
2022 年 9 月

Table of Contents

目　　录

第一章　抗肿瘤疗法导言　001

第二章　痤疮样皮疹　020

第三章　毛发疾病　027

第四章　光敏和光反应　039

第五章　角化过度性反应　053

第六章　硬化性皮疹　073

第七章　手足反应　082

第八章　抗肿瘤治疗的口腔黏膜反应　096

第九章　化疗引起的甲反应　125

第十章　新生物反应　134

第十一章　过敏和荨麻疹　147

第十二章　干燥、瘙痒和裂隙　154

第十三章　放射性皮炎　157

第一章

抗肿瘤疗法导言

詹妮弗·吴(Jennifer Wu),马里奥·拉库蒂尔(Mario E. Lacouture)

盛友渔 张 波 译

一 概述:肿瘤发病率和系统抗肿瘤治疗的类型

在过去的几十年里,肿瘤治疗发生了革命性的变化,每年都有许多抗肿瘤新疗法被开发出来,并被批准用于多种类型的肿瘤[1]。根据世界卫生组织(WHO)的数据,每年有超过1 000万人被确诊为肿瘤,以及有800万肿瘤相关死亡病例和3 000万肿瘤幸存者[2]。随着发病率和病死率的增加,肿瘤的预防和治疗已成为公共卫生的一个重要问题。然而,随着新的治疗方式和联合治疗方案的迅速出现以及患者生存期的延长,抗肿瘤治疗不良事件的发生率也在增加。不同的抗肿瘤治疗方式,如细胞毒性化疗、靶向治疗、免疫检查点抑制剂(immune checkpoint inhibitor,ICI)、放疗、过继性T淋巴细胞治疗和造血干细胞移植,都有不同的皮肤不良事件(adverse events,AE)谱,可能涉及皮肤、头发、指甲和黏膜。皮肤不良事件不仅损害患者的身体功能和生活质量,还可导致用药剂量减少、方案修正和抗肿瘤治疗的中断,最终对肿瘤预后造成负面甚至危及生命的影响[3]。了解与抗肿瘤治疗相关的皮肤不良事件的流行病学和临床表现,有助于早期识别及时、适当地处理,这对继续抗肿瘤治疗、改善预后和维持生活质量非常重要。因此,强烈建议在开始抗肿瘤治疗之前,告知患者一些潜在的皮肤不良事件以及预防和处理的策略。本章旨在简要介绍抗肿瘤治疗及其相关的皮肤不良反应事件(图1-1,表1-1、1-2)。以下章节将逐一讨论各种类型的皮肤表现。

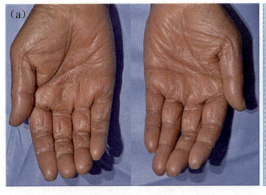
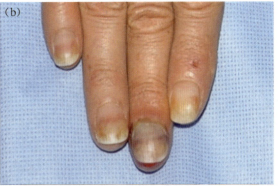

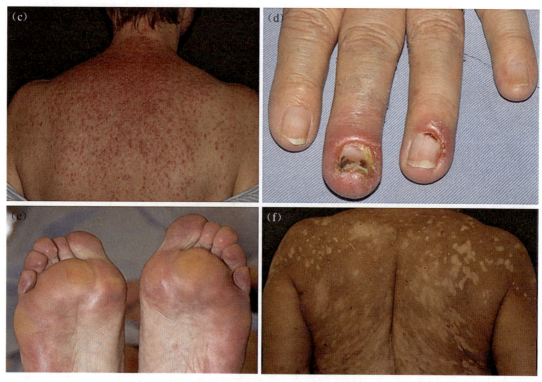

图 1-1 抗肿瘤治疗的皮肤不良事件

(a)卡培他滨诱发的手足综合征(hand-foot syndrome, HFS);(b)多西他赛相关的指尖肿胀、甲下出血和甲剥离症;(c)表皮生长因子受体抑制剂(epidermal growth factor receptor inhibitor, EGFRI)相关的丘疹脓疱性皮疹;(d)表皮生长因子受体抑制剂相关的甲沟炎;(e)多靶点激酶抑制剂(multitargeted kinase inhibitor, MKI)相关的手足皮肤反应(hand-foot skin reaction, HFSR);(f)免疫检查点抑制剂诱发的白癜风样皮损。

表 1-1 抗肿瘤治疗及其相关的皮肤不良事件汇总

系统抗肿瘤治疗类型	皮肤不良事件	常见的致病药物(发生率%)
	手足综合征,又称掌跖感觉丧失性红斑(palmar-plantar erythrodysesthesia, PPE)综合征	卡培他滨(43%~63%),持续输注5-氟尿嘧啶、阿糖胞苷、多西他赛(5%~10%)、多柔比星(阿霉素)和脂质体多柔比星(pegylated liposomal doxorubicin, PLD)(45%)
	速发型过敏反应(immediate hypersensitivity reaction, IHSR)	紫杉烷类(30%,如不包括前驱用药)、铂类为基础的化疗方案(12%~24%)[21]
	外渗反应(extravasation reactions)	刺激物:铂基烷基化剂、紫杉烷类和拓扑异构酶抑制剂 起疱剂:蒽环类、长春花碱和氮芥(0.1%~6%)[17,22]
	色素改变	白消安、环磷酰胺、异环磷酰胺、博来霉素、5-氟尿嘧啶、长春瑞滨、福莫司汀、多西他赛等

(续表)

系统抗肿瘤治疗类型	皮肤不良事件		常见的致病药物（发生率%）
	甲营养不良	博氏线（Beau line）	博来霉素、顺铂、多西他赛、多柔比星、美法仑和长春新碱
		甲剥离	米托蒽醌、多西他赛、蒽环类药物和紫杉醇
	化疗所致脱发（chemotherapy-induced alopecia，CIA）		
	化疗所致急性可逆性脱发		紫杉烷类是最常引起CIA的药物之一[33,34]
	化疗所致持久性脱发（chemotherapy induced persistent alopecia，CIPAL）		白消安、噻替哌、氟尿嘧啶+表柔比星+环磷酰胺（FEC方案）和紫杉烷类
	放疗回忆反应		多柔比星、紫杉烷类、5-氟尿嘧啶、吉西他滨和卡培他滨有最多报道[44]
表皮生长因子受体抑制剂（EGFRI）	丘疹脓疱性皮疹（papulopustular eruption，PPE）或痤疮样皮疹		EGFRI用于治疗晚期或转移性非小细胞肺癌（如阿法替尼、厄洛替尼、吉非替尼、耐昔妥珠单抗）、胰腺癌（如厄洛替尼）、乳腺癌（如拉帕替尼、奈拉替尼）、结肠癌（如西妥昔单抗、帕尼单抗）、头颈癌（如西妥昔单抗），以及基于肿瘤个体突变的更广泛临床应用[23,49,54]
	色素改变		
	发质改变，非瘢痕性脱发和瘢痕性脱发，面部多毛症和睫毛粗长症		
	甲沟炎		
	鼻前庭炎（nasal vestibulitis，NV）		
多靶点激酶抑制剂（MKI）	手足皮肤反应（HFSR）		索拉非尼（多吉美）和舒尼替尼（索坦）（9%~62%的患者使用索拉非尼和舒尼替尼、瑞戈非尼、阿西替尼、帕唑帕尼）
BRAF抑制剂（BRAF inhibitor，BRAFI）	非恶性角化过度皮疹		维莫非尼和达拉非尼
	皮肤鳞状细胞癌（squamous cell carcinoma，SCC）		
	光敏性		
	斑丘疹、丘疹脓疱性皮疹伴或不伴瘙痒的毛囊中心性皮疹[53]，在四肢近端、躯干和面部的毛周角化样皮疹（5%~9%）[79]，手足皮肤反应[80]		
MEK抑制剂			曲美替尼、考比替尼
BRAF抑制剂联合MEK抑制剂			

(续表)

系统抗肿瘤治疗类型	皮肤不良事件	常见的致病药物（发生率%）
Hedgehog信号通路抑制剂	脱发,毛囊性皮炎,过敏反应,角化棘皮瘤和皮肤鳞状细胞癌	维莫德吉、索尼德吉
免疫检查点抑制剂	皮疹,瘙痒,白癜风	免疫检查点抑制剂：CTLA4抗体、PD-1抗体和PD-L1抗体
	自身免疫性大疱性皮肤病	PD-1抗体和PD-L1抗体
	严重皮肤不良反应(severe cutaneous adverse reaction, SCAR)	CTLA4抗体、PD1抗体和PD-L1抗体
嵌合抗原受体T细胞免疫疗法(chimeric antigen receptor-modified T lymphocytes therapy, CAR-T)	皮疹[细胞因子释放综合征（cytokine releasing syndrome, CRS)]	嵌合抗原受体T细胞免疫治疗
放疗	放射性皮炎(radiation dermatitis, RD)	电离辐射
造血干细胞移植(hematopoietic stem cell transplantation, HSCT)	皮肤移植物抗宿主病(graft-versus-host disease, GVHD)	造血干细胞移植
肿瘤治疗的其他皮肤不良反应	与抗肿瘤治疗相关的皮肤感染[63]	
	Stevens-Johnson综合征/中毒性表皮坏死松解症(Stevens-Johnson syndrome/toxic epidermal necrolysis, SJS/TEN)	SJS：苯达莫司汀 TEN：苯达莫司汀、白消安、苯丁酸氮芥、氟达拉滨、洛莫司汀和甲基苄肼[美国食品药品监督管理局(food and drug administration, FDA)不良事件报告系统]

表1-2 抗肿瘤治疗相关皮肤不良事件通用术语标准(common terminology criteria for adverse events, CTCAE)分级

不良事件	分级				
	1	2	3	4	5
严重度	轻度	中度	严重或医学意义重大,但不立即危及生命	危及生命	死亡
描述	无症状或症状轻;只需临床或诊断性观察;不需要干预	最低限度、局部或非侵袭性干预;限制特定年龄的工具性日常生活活动[a]	住院治疗或延长住院治疗;影响日常生活自理活动[b]	需要采取紧急干预措施	不良事件相关的死亡

(续表)

不良事件	分级				
	1	2	3	4	5
手足综合征(HFS)(掌跖感觉丧失性红斑):一种以手掌或足底皮肤发红、明显不适、肿胀和刺痛为特征的疾病	轻微的皮肤变化或皮炎(如红斑、水肿或角化过度),无疼痛	皮肤变化(如脱屑、水疱、出血、水肿或角化过度),伴有疼痛;影响工具性日常生活活动	严重的皮肤变化(如脱屑、水疱、出血、水肿或角化过度),伴有疼痛;影响日常生活自理活动		
痤疮样皮疹:一种以丘疹和脓疱性皮疹为特征的疾病,通常累及面部、头皮、上胸部和背部	丘疹和/或脓疱<10%体表面积,伴或不伴瘙痒或压痛	丘疹和/或脓疱占10%~30%体表面积,伴或不伴瘙痒或压痛;伴有心理社会影响;影响工具性日常生活活动	丘疹和/或脓疱>30%体表面积,伴或不伴瘙痒或压痛;影响日常生活自理活动;伴局部重复感染,需口服抗生素	累及任何体表面积范围的丘疹和/或脓疱,伴或不伴瘙痒或压痛;影响日常生活自理活动;伴广泛的重复感染,需静脉滴注抗生素;危及生命	死亡
斑丘疹皮疹:一种以斑疹(扁平)和丘疹(隆起)为特征的疾病,又称麻疹样皮疹,是最常见的皮肤不良事件之一,常累及躯干上部,向心性扩散,并伴有瘙痒	斑疹/丘疹<10%体表面积,伴或不伴主观症状(如瘙痒、烧灼感、紧绷感)	斑疹/丘疹占10%~30%体表面积,伴或不伴主观症状(如瘙痒、烧灼感、紧绷感);影响工具性日常生活活动	斑疹/丘疹>30%体表面积,伴或不伴主观症状;影响日常生活自理活动		
瘙痒症:一种以皮肤强烈的瘙痒感为特征的疾病	轻度或局限性;局部治疗	强烈或广泛;间歇性;皮肤因擦伤而变化(如水肿、丘疹、脱屑、苔藓样变、渗出/结痂);口服药物干预;影响工具性日常生活活动	强烈或广泛;持续性;影响日常生活自理活动和睡眠;需口服糖皮质激素或免疫抑制剂		

(续表)

不良事件	分级				
	1	2	3	4	5
皮肤干燥:一种以皮肤片状和暗沉为特征的疾病;毛孔通常很细;纹理像纸质样薄	<10%体表面积,无红斑或瘙痒	占10%~30%体表面积,伴有红斑或瘙痒;影响工具性日常生活活动	>30%体表面积,伴瘙痒;影响日常生活自理活动		
光敏:一种以皮肤对光的敏感性增加为特征的疾病	无痛性红斑,红斑<10%体表面积	疼痛性红斑,占10%~30%体表面积	红斑>30%体表面积或伴水疱;光敏;需口服糖皮质激素;止痛治疗(如麻醉药或非甾体类抗炎药)	危及生命;需要采取紧急干预措施	
脱发:一种以在特定的年龄和身体部位,与正常人相比头发密度降低为特征的疾病	头发脱落<50%正常发量,从远处看不明显,仅在近距离检查时明显;可能需要通过改变发型来掩盖脱发,但不需要假发或发片来遮饰	头发脱落≥50%正常发量,发量与其他健康人明显不同;需要使用假发或发片才能完全遮饰脱发区域;伴有心理社会影响			
手足皮肤反应(HFSR):一种以手掌或足底发红、明显不适、肿胀和刺痛为特征的疾病	轻微皮肤变化或皮炎(如红斑、水肿或角化过度),无疼痛	皮肤变化(如剥脱、水疱、出血、水肿或角化过度),伴疼痛;影响工具性日常生活活动	严重的皮肤变化(如脱屑、水疱、出血、水肿或角化过度),伴有疼痛;影响日常生活自理活动	—	—
放射性皮炎	轻微红斑或干性脱屑	中度活跃的红斑;片状潮湿脱屑,主要分布于皮肤皱褶部位;中度水肿	潮湿脱屑,不仅限于皮肤皱褶部位;轻度创伤或摩擦引起出血	皮肤坏死或全层皮肤破溃;受累部位自发性出血	

来源:改编自不良事件通用术语标准(CTCAE):https://evs.nci.nih.gov/ftp1/CTCAE/CTCAE_4.03_2010-06-14_QuickReference_5x7.pdf。

注意:一字线(—)代表分级不适用。并非所有分级都适合任何不良事件,因此有些不良事件少于5个分级。5级(死亡)不适用于一些不良事件。

a:工具性日常生活活动,指烹饪、购物、打电话、处理财务等。

b:日常生活自理活动,指自己洗澡、穿衣和脱衣,自己进食、上厕所、吃药,无卧病不起。

二 抗肿瘤治疗及其相关的皮肤不良事件

(一) 细胞毒化疗

1. 化疗中毒性红斑

化疗中毒性红斑(toxic erythema of chemotherapy,TEC)描述了因化疗引起的复合性皮肤毒性反应,由可重复的非免疫介导效应所诱发。TEC 的临床特征是腋窝、腹股沟、手足以及较少发生于肘部、膝盖和耳部的红斑或斑块,伴有疼痛、灼烧感、感觉异常和瘙痒。TEC 通常在应用化疗药物后的几天至 3 周内出现,但在接受低剂量、持续输注 5-氟尿嘧啶(5-FU)或口服制剂的患者中,可能会在 2~10 个月出现。受累区域可见大疱和糜烂。皮损通常是自限性的,但在再次使用相同药物后可能复发[4]。手足综合征(HFS)是 TEC 的一个亚型,主要累及手掌和足底[4,5]。与 TEC 相关的化疗药物通常包括阿糖胞苷(Ara-C)、蒽环类药物、多柔比星、脂质体多柔比星(PLD)、5-氟尿嘧啶、卡培他滨(5-氟尿嘧啶前体药物)、紫杉烷类药物(多西他赛和紫杉醇)和甲氨蝶呤。博来霉素、白消安、卡莫司汀、洛莫司汀、顺铂、卡铂、氯法拉滨、环磷酰胺、异环磷酰胺、依托泊苷、吉西他滨、羟基脲(hydroyurea,HU)、美法仑、6-巯基嘌呤、米托蒽醌、酪氨酸激酶抑制剂(伊马替尼、舒尼替尼)、替加氟、噻替哌和长春瑞滨也与 TEC 有关。

2. 手足综合征

手足综合征(HFS)曾被称为掌跖感觉丧失性红斑,是一种由某些化疗药物[4,5]引起的皮肤不良事件,最常见的是卡培他滨、5-氟尿嘧啶、阿糖胞苷、紫杉烷类、多柔比星和脂质体多柔比星[6-10]。HFS 表现为感觉障碍,随后手掌和足底出现对称性疼痛性红斑和水肿。皮损可能发展为水疱、结痂或溃疡[10,11]。HFS 的病理生理学机制尚不完全清楚,但认为与细胞毒性化疗药物或代谢物累积诱导的角质形成细胞凋亡有关,药物代谢物可能通过汗液在手掌和足底排泄增多[12-14]。也有报道环氧化酶-2(COX-2)过度表达介导的炎症过程参与发病机制[15]。HFS 明显影响患者的生活质量,限制日常活动,并且经常需要调整药物剂量甚至停止化疗[16]。

3. 急性过敏反应

速发型过敏反应(IHSR)通常发生在开始的两个化疗周期输注期间或输注后不久,发病迅速,在几分钟内发作[17]。临床表现各异,包括非特异性斑丘疹、荨麻疹、血管性水肿、面部潮红和瘙痒,伴或不伴低血压、呼吸困难或发冷等全身症状和体征[17,18]。IHSR 可表现为危及生命的过敏性休克,需要临床注意防范。

紫杉烷类(多西他赛和紫杉醇)是最常引起 IHSR 的药物,如果没有(化疗)前驱药,IHSR 发生率为 30%。紫杉烷类已被批准并经常用于治疗转移性或局部晚期乳腺癌、非小细胞肺癌、前列腺癌、胃癌、头颈癌和卵巢癌[1,17-19]。潜在的机制被认为与紫杉醇(Cremophor EL®,蓖麻油载体)溶剂的过敏反应有关,而多西他赛(吐温 80,聚氧乙烯-20-山梨醇单油酸酯)的溶剂较少引起[20]。在 12%~24%的患者中也观察到铂类药物诱发的 IHSR[21]。

4. 外渗反应

接受化疗的患者中有 0.1%～6% 可发生外渗反应。严重程度因化疗药物的剂量、浓度和类型而异。致病药物包括刺激剂（如铂基烷基化剂、紫杉烷类和拓扑异构酶抑制剂）和起疱剂（如蒽环类、长春花生物碱和氮芥）[17,22]。刺激剂通常引起较轻的炎症反应，表现为红斑、水肿和疼痛。起疱剂可导致更严重的反应，包括水疱形成、溃疡和组织坏死[23]。

5. 色素改变

烷基化剂如氮芥（环磷酰胺、异环磷酰胺）、烷基磺酸盐（白消安）和亚硝基脲类（福莫司汀）通常会导致皮肤、黏膜色素沉着。博来霉素、5-氟尿嘧啶、长春瑞滨和多西他赛也可引起色素沉着。这些皮肤问题通常会自发缓解，可能不需要停止化疗[24]。环磷酰胺和异环磷酰胺可能导致指甲、手掌和足底的局部色素沉着[25,26]，而白消安可能导致艾迪生病（Addison disease）样全身性皮肤色素沉着。博来霉素治疗的患者中有 20% 出现特征性鞭毛状色素沉着[27,28]。蛇形静脉色素沉着与 5-氟尿嘧啶、长春瑞滨、福莫司汀和多西他赛相关[29,30]。

6. 毛发和甲改变

（1）甲毒性　据报道，包括紫杉烷类（46%）、脂质体多柔比星（7%）、蒽环类药物（19%）、拓扑替康（14%）和其他药物（14%）在内的化疗药物的皮肤、指甲和毛发不良反应的总发生率为 86.8%，其中 23.1% 出现甲改变[6]。细胞毒性化疗药物会破坏指甲基质，导致甲板出现横向隆起，即博氏线，这通常是自限性的[31]。甲床受累时会发生甲剥离。疼痛、甲沟炎、肉芽组织生长、甲脱落和继发性细菌感染伴脓肿形成可能使甲分离复杂化，从而影响患者的日常活动和生活质量[32]。与化疗相关的常见甲改变还包括甲脆化、变色、裂片形出血、甲下血肿和色素沉着[32]。

（2）化疗所致脱发　据统计，65% 接受化疗的患者出现化疗所致的脱发（chemotherapy-induced alopecia，CIA）。47% 的女性患者认为 CIA 是化疗最具创伤性的影响[33]。紫杉烷类包括多西他赛、紫杉醇和蒽环类药物是最常见的诱发药物[33-36]。CIA 的风险因素包括长期治疗、高剂量或多次暴露[33,37]。

1）化疗所致可逆性脱发：生长期脱发是化疗诱导的急性可逆性脱发的常见原因，通常发生在前 4 个治疗周期之后[37]。任何毛发区域，包括头皮、睫毛、眉毛、胡须、腋毛、阴毛和体毛都可受累。化疗结束后 3～6 个月可见到毛发再生；然而，1/3 的患者可能会经历头发再生量减少以及发质、发色改变[35]。

2）持续性化疗所致脱发（persistent chemotherapy-induced alopecia，pCIA）：是指停止化疗后≥6 个月的头发再生不完全或缺失[34]。pCIA 通常表现为弥漫性脱发或头发稀疏，顶部区域更为明显，临床特征类似于雄激素性脱发[35,38-42]。睫毛、眉毛、腋毛、阴毛和体毛也可受累[39,40,43]。据报道，白消安、噻替哌、氟尿嘧啶+表柔比星+环磷酰胺（FEC 方案）和紫杉烷类药物可引起 pCIA[39,40,42]。Kluger 等人估计接受多西他赛治疗的患者 pCIA 的发病率约为 2%，但这个结果被认为是低估了[39]。pCIA 的病理机制尚不清楚，推测是由于基质细胞从毛乳头中分离，以及紫杉烷类对毛母质角质形成细胞或毛囊隆突干细胞有直接的细胞毒性作用所致[34,39,40]。

(二) 放疗回忆反应

放疗回忆反应(radiation recall)是一种急性炎症反应,限于化疗引发的先前放疗区域。多柔比星、紫杉烷类、5-氟尿嘧啶、吉西他滨和卡培他滨最常与放疗回忆反应现象相关[44]。发病率根据药物各异,为1.8%～11.5%[23,45,46]。放疗回忆反应的潜伏期从几个月到几年[45,46]。虽然发病机制尚不清楚,但细胞毒性化疗诱导的记忆细胞介导的过敏反应可能发挥作用[44,47]。

(三) 肿瘤的靶向治疗

靶向治疗通过抑制在肿瘤生长中具有核心作用的特定信号通路,实现抗肿瘤效果,包括表皮生长因子受体(EGFR)和细胞内丝裂原活化蛋白激酶(mitogen-activated protein kinase,MAPK)或 RAS-RAF-MEK-MAPK 信号通路[48,49]。肿瘤靶向治疗的皮肤不良事件与细胞毒性化疗不同。然而,仍存在导致药物减量、抗肿瘤治疗中断和生活质量受损的可能,并将影响临床预后[50]。因此,全面了解这些皮肤不良事件的预防、诊断和处理至关重要。靶向 EGFR 或血管内皮生长因子受体(vascular endothelial growth factor receptor,VEGFR)信号通路的酪氨酸激酶抑制剂(TKI)的皮肤不良事件已被很好地阐述,其发生率和严重程度取决于特定的靶向治疗和不同的剂量[23,51-54]。与靶向治疗相关的常见皮肤不良事件包括痤疮样皮疹、手足皮肤反应、干燥症、瘙痒症、黏膜炎、脱发、皮肤赘生物、色素改变以及毛发和甲病变[50]。

1. 表皮生长因子受体抑制剂

表皮生长因子受体抑制剂(EGFRI)基于肿瘤的个体突变已在临床广泛使用,包括晚期或转移性非小细胞肺癌(吉非替尼、厄洛替尼、阿法替尼、奥希替尼、耐昔妥珠单抗)、胰腺癌(厄洛替尼)、乳腺癌(拉帕替尼、奈拉替尼)、结肠癌(西妥昔单抗、帕尼单抗)和头颈癌(西妥昔单抗)[23,49,54]。皮肤毒性反应是最常见的 EGFRI 相关不良事件,可表现为丘疹脓疱疹(丘疹脓疱性皮疹、痤疮样皮疹)、干燥症、瘙痒症,头发、指甲和甲周异常[23,51,52,55]。这些皮肤不良事件可能引起疼痛和衰弱,并对治疗强度、患者的日常生活和生活质量产生负面影响[56]。

(1) 丘疹脓疱性皮疹或痤疮样皮疹　痤疮样皮疹是 EGFRI 治疗中最常见的皮肤不良事件,90%以上的患者受到影响[55]。EGFRI 不仅抑制癌细胞的特定信号通路,也干扰正常组织中的信号转导,如表皮角质形成细胞、皮脂腺、毛囊上皮和甲周组织,导致皮肤毒性[23,51,54]。丘疹脓疱性皮疹主要表现为皮脂溢出区域(面部、头皮和躯干上部)的痤疮样毛囊,毛囊周围丘疹和无菌性脓疱,通常伴有干燥症、瘙痒,甚至疼痛[57,58]。皮疹通常是短暂的,出现在最初的几周内;然而,即使在停止治疗后,干燥症、瘙痒、炎症后红斑或色素沉着也可能持续存在[56,59]。据报道,EGFRI 皮肤毒性的发生与良好的癌症预后相关[60]。荟萃分析显示,在非小细胞肺癌患者中,皮疹的出现与死亡率降低60%以及疾病进展风险降低55%相关[60,61]。

(2) 色素改变　系统回顾显示,靶向治疗引起皮肤和头发色素改变的总发生率分别为17.7%和21.5%。据报道,EGFRI 和伊马替尼是最常见的原因[62]。

(3) 毛发和甲改变 甲沟炎,即甲周红斑、肿胀、疼痛,伴或不伴甲周化脓性肉芽肿样损害,可在 EGFRI 治疗开始 2～3 个月后发生,不同 EGFRI 中其发病率为 12%～58%[52,63]。皮损最初是无菌性的,但可以合并感染[23]。可能的机制是角质形成细胞损伤和细胞因子失调引起的甲周炎症,嵌甲和局部创伤可能加剧这种影响[23]。毛发改变可见头发质地和颜色的变化、非瘢痕性脱发、面部多毛症和睫毛粗长症。

2. 哺乳动物雷帕霉素靶蛋白抑制剂

雷帕霉素信号通路的磷脂酰肌醇-3-激酶(PI3K)、Akt、哺乳动物雷帕霉素靶蛋白(mammalian target of rapamycin, mTOR)在多种恶性肿瘤中上调。mTOR 抑制剂(如替西罗莫司和依维莫司)的皮肤不良事件很常见,如口腔炎、皮疹和甲改变(如甲沟炎)。据报道,44%的患者出现 mTOR 抑制剂相关口腔炎。与化疗相关口腔炎不同的是,mTOR 抑制剂相关口腔炎表现为非角化上皮上的散在性口疮[64]。1/3 的患者可出现皮疹,通常表现为斑丘疹或丘疹脓疱,类似 EGFRI 诱发的丘疹脓疱性皮疹[64],这被认为与抑制 PI3K-Akt-mTOR 信号通路有关,PI3K-Akt-mTOR 信号通路是 EGFR 的下游效应通路之一[50]。

3. 多靶点激酶抑制剂

多靶点激酶抑制剂(MKI)如伊马替尼、索拉非尼、舒尼替尼、瑞戈非尼、阿西替尼和帕唑帕尼,通过干扰参与细胞生长和血管生成的分子信号通路实现抗癌作用[65]。皮肤不良事件最常见于应用 MKI 的患者,由于这些靶向信号通路的共性,临床特征重叠[23,66,67]。

(1) 手足皮肤反应 手足皮肤反应(HFSR)是最常见的皮肤不良事件之一,发生于 9%～62% 接受 MKI 治疗的患者中,如索拉非尼、舒尼替尼、瑞戈非尼、阿西替尼和帕唑帕尼[48,65,68-75]。HFSR 的特征性表现是对称性肢端红斑,伴有脱屑和裂隙,随后出现角化过度(表现为足底受压区被红斑/水肿围绕的浅黄色疼痛斑块),偶尔形成水疱[68]。HFSR 的机制包括手掌和足底的直接压力和摩擦导致水疱和毛细血管内皮损伤;通过抑制 VEGFR 和血小板衍生生长因子受体(platelet-derived growth factor receptor, PDGFR)影响内皮愈合;对角质形成细胞的直接细胞毒性作用和 Fas-FasL 信号通路失调相关[48,65,71]。

4. BRAF 抑制剂

BRAF 是一种丝氨酸-苏氨酸蛋白激酶,在调节细胞增殖、分化、迁移、存活和凋亡的 RAS-RAF-MEK-MAPK 信号通路中发挥作用[48,53,76,77]。BRAF 在 40%～60% 的皮肤黑色素瘤中发生突变,是人类癌症中最常见的突变蛋白激酶之一,包括毛细胞白血病、甲状腺乳头状癌、浆液性卵巢癌、结直肠癌和前列腺癌[64]。皮肤不良事件是与使用维莫非尼和达拉非尼相关的最重要和最常见的不良事件之一,发生于高达 95% 的患者[77,78],其明显的特征包括斑丘疹、光敏、角化过度皮损或皮肤肿瘤[53]。野生型 *BRAF* 细胞或含有 *RAS* 突变细胞的反常激活可增强 MAPK 途径的活性,从而导致角质形成、细胞增殖或肿瘤形成[53,76,77]。

(1) 皮疹 皮疹是最常见的皮肤不良事件,影响 64%～75% 接受 BRAF 抑制剂治疗的患者,维莫非尼比达拉非尼更常见。在接受 BRAF 抑制剂治疗的患者中可以看到各种皮疹,包括近端肢体、躯干和面部(5%～9%)的斑丘疹、丘疹脓疱疹或毛周角化样皮疹[79];伴或不伴瘙痒的毛囊中心性皮疹[53],以及手足皮肤反应[80]。皮疹通常在开始治疗后 2 周内发生。

(2) 光敏 光敏(photosensitivity)是一种众所周知的不良事件,30%～52% 接受维莫非尼治疗的患者会出现,表现为急性红斑、烧灼感和疼痛性水疱,好发于日光暴露部位[53]。

(3) 非恶性角化过度皮疹　鳞状增生/角质形成细胞性皮疹发生于60%~85%接受BRAFI治疗的患者。疣状角化病是60%以上患者最常见的表现,通常在治疗过程中的几周内出现[53,76,77]。其他病变包括手掌/足底压力摩擦点角化过度(40%)、皮肤乳头状瘤、寻常疣、脂溢性角化病(seborrheic keratoses,SK)、疣状角化不良瘤、炎症性光化性角化病(actinic keratosis,AK)和角化棘皮瘤(keratoacanthoma,KA)[53]。

(4) 皮肤鳞状细胞癌　皮肤鳞状细胞癌(SCC)通常为角化棘皮瘤型,在皮肤曝光区域(4%~36%)表现为快速生长的圆顶状火山口样结节[53,76,77],通常在维莫非尼等BRAFI治疗后早期出现,中位发病时间为8周[53]。

5. MEK抑制剂

EGFR、*RAS*或*BRAF*水平的上游突变可驱动RAS-RAF-MEK-MAPK信号通路内的组成性激活,使MEK蛋白聚集导致肿瘤生长[64]。MEK抑制剂(MEKI)如曲美替尼和考比替尼的皮肤不良事件与EGFRI相似,包括丘疹脓疱性皮疹(PPE)、干燥症、瘙痒症、脱发、甲沟炎、色素沉着、睫毛粗长症、毛发质地变化和面部多毛症。PPE是MEKI最常见的皮肤不良事件,发生于52%~93%的患者中。受累皮肤的继发性细菌感染并不少见[77,81]。

6. BRAF抑制剂联合MEK抑制剂

由于下游MEK抑制对BRAF抑制剂反常激活MAPK通路的影响,BRAF抑制剂联合MEK抑制剂治疗似乎比单独使用BRAF抑制剂的皮肤毒性状况有所改善[64]。

与单独使用达拉非尼相比,达拉非尼与曲美替尼联合使用,可显著降低皮肤鳞状细胞癌(0% *vs.* 26.1%)、疣状角化病和短暂性棘层松解皮肤病(Grover病)的发病率,但毛囊炎的发生率更高(40% *vs.* 6.7%)[76,77,82,83]。

7. Hedgehog信号通路抑制剂(维莫德吉、索尼德吉)

Hedgehog信号通路异常激活是基底细胞癌(basal cell carcinoma,BCC)发病机制中的关键驱动因素。维莫德吉和索尼德吉是Hedgehog信号通路的小分子抑制剂,被批准用于治疗成人转移性BCC或部分患者的局部晚期BCC。常见的不良反应包括肌肉痉挛、味觉缺失/嗅觉障碍、脱发、体重减轻和疲劳[84]。脱发是Hedgehog信号通路抑制剂常见的一种皮肤不良事件,46%~66%的患者受到影响,与细胞毒性化疗相比发病相对延迟,在治疗2个月后发生[84-87]。其机制可能与Hedgehog信号通路在正常毛囊周期中的重要作用有关。毛囊毒性,如脱发和毛囊炎,被推测可能为肿瘤反应的替代标识[85]。毛囊性皮炎、过敏反应、角化棘皮瘤和皮肤鳞状细胞癌作为Hedgehog信号通路抑制剂的皮肤不良事件也有报道[84-91]。

(四) 免疫检查点抑制剂

细胞毒性T淋巴细胞抗原-4(cytotoxic T lymphocyte antigen-4,CTLA-4)信号通路和程序性细胞死亡受体-1(PD-1)/PD配体-1(PD-L1)信号通路是免疫稳态和肿瘤诱导免疫抑制的免疫检查点[92]。由于免疫检查点抑制剂(ICI)通过中断肿瘤细胞诱导的抑制信号和免疫逃逸机制来恢复抗肿瘤免疫,它们可能同时诱导各种器官系统的自身免疫和炎症,最常见的是皮肤、胃肠道、内分泌腺和肝脏,称为免疫相关不良事件(immune-related adverse event，irAE）[93-95]。皮肤 irAE 的确切发病机制仍未阐明。可能的机制包括 T 细胞对肿瘤和健康组织中共同抗原的活性增加，例如白癜风；先前存在的自身抗体水平增加，例如大疱性类天疱疮（bullous pemphigoid，BP）；炎症细胞因子水平增加，例如银屑病和银屑病样皮疹[95]。

1. 瘙痒、皮疹和白癜风

皮肤 irAE 是 ICI 最早和最常见的不良事件之一，包括瘙痒、皮疹和白癜风。白癜风多见于黑色素瘤患者[94,96-98]。自身免疫性大疱性皮病[99]、苔藓样皮炎/黏膜炎、银屑病加重、银屑病样皮疹、斑秃/普秃、重症多形[性]红斑（Stevens-Johnson 综合征）和中毒性表皮坏死松解症（TEN）也被报道是 ICI 相关皮肤不良事件[93,98,100-104]。越来越多的证据表明，ICI 治疗期间出现白癜风和/或皮疹与良好的临床预后相关[92,103,105-107]。

2. 大疱性类天疱疮

大疱性类天疱疮（BP）可能在接受抗 PD-1/PD-L1 治疗的患者中发生，被认为由 T 细胞和 B 细胞免疫介导所致[99,108]。与 ICI 相关的 BP 可能在 ICI 开始后的数月内发生，伴有或先有瘙痒，并可能在停止治疗后持续存在。皮肤活检、直接和间接免疫荧光检测以及血清自身抗体（BP180 抗体、BP230 抗体）测定有助于诊断[99]。

3. 严重皮肤不良反应

严重皮肤不良反应（SCAR）很少见，但有文献报道了与 ICI 相关的重症多形[性]红斑（Stevens-Johnson 综合征）、中毒性表皮坏死松解症（TEN）、伴嗜酸性粒细胞增多和系统症状的药疹（drug reaction with eosinophilia and systemic symptoms，DRESS）[109-111]。对临床和用药史进行全面检查有助于准确诊断和判断致敏药物。

（五）嵌合抗原受体 T 细胞治疗

过继性细胞治疗是一种有效且有前景的肿瘤治疗方法。在给予嵌合抗原受体（chimeric antigen receptor T cell therapy，CAR）T 细胞治疗后，可以很快出现细胞因子释放综合征（cytokine release syndrome，CRS）[92]。当靶向蛋白质的 T 细胞受体（T-cell receptor，TCR）在正常组织中表达时，可能会发生由给药 T 细胞诱导的自身免疫反应。例如，当源自黑色素细胞的蛋白质被识别 T 细胞 1 黑色素瘤抗原（MART-1）和糖蛋白 100（gp100）的 TCR 靶向时，会发生皮肤、眼和内耳毒性[92]。

（六）放疗

放射性皮炎通常发生在放疗开始后 2～3 周[112]。急性放射性皮炎通常表现为红斑、干性或湿性脱屑和溃疡，具有自限性，通常在 2～3 个月后消退。晚期毒性通常发生在治疗过程的后期，间隔>90 天。皮损包括毛细血管扩张、萎缩、纤维化、水肿和溃疡，皮损可能持续存在并对患者的生活质量造成持久的负面影响[55,112,113]。

（七）造血干细胞移植

移植物抗宿主病（graft-versus-host disease，GVHD）是同种异体造血干细胞移植（allogeneic hematopoietic stem cell transplant，allo-HSCT）受者的主要并发症，发病率

为 40%～60%,在与治疗相关死亡中占 15%[114,115]。皮肤 GVHD 最常见,60%～80%的患者受到影响,可导致长期并发症,包括美容方面、功能性甚至危及生命的后遗症[114,115]。皮肤 GVHD 的特征性表现为皮肤异色病、扁平苔藓样疹、硬化萎缩性苔癣样皮损、硬斑病样硬化和深部硬化或筋膜炎[114]。

三 结语

肿瘤的维持治疗对患者生存至关重要。新疗法的迅速发展带来了有希望的抗肿瘤疗效以及各种不良事件。皮肤不良事件是最常见的,可能严重影响患者的生活质量。越来越多的证据表明,通过全面的治疗前评估、先期治疗、早期诊断和适当处理,这些皮肤不良事件是可以预防和控制的。皮肤科医生在减少皮肤不良事件的影响方面发挥着关键作用。早期、及时的皮肤科会诊和包括皮肤科医生在内的多学科团队有利于优化肿瘤的治疗。

参 考 文 献

1. Giavina-Bianchi P, Patil SU, Banerji A. Immediate hypersensitivity reaction to chemotherapeutic agents. *J Allergy Clin Immunol Pract* 2017;5(3):593-9.
2. Santoni M et al. Risk of pruritus in cancer patients treated with biological therapies: A systematic review and meta-analysis of clinical trials. *Crit Rev Oncol Hematol* 2015;96(2):206-19.
3. Lacouture ME. Management of dermatologic toxicities. *JNCCN* 2015;13(5 Suppl):686-9.
4. Bolognia JL, Cooper DL, Glusac EJ. Toxic erythema of chemotherapy: A useful clinical term. *J Am Acad Dermatol* 2008;59(3):524-9.
5. Parker TL, Cooper DL, Seropian SE, Bolognia JL. Toxic erythema of chemotherapy following i.v. BU plus fludarabine for allogeneic PBSC transplant. *Bone Marrow Transplant* 2013;48(5):646-50.
6. Hackbarth M, Haas N, Fotopoulou C, Lichtenegger W, Sehouli J. Chemotherapy-induced dermatological toxicity: Frequencies and impact on quality of life in women's cancers. Results of a prospective study. *Support Care Cancer* 2008;16(3):267-73.
7. Saif MW, Katirtzoglou NA, Syrigos KN. Capecitabine: An overview of the side effects and their management. *Anti-Cancer Drugs* 2008;19(5):447-64.
8. Chew L, Chuen VS. Cutaneous reaction associated with weekly docetaxel administration. *J Oncol Pharm Pract: ISOPP* 2009;15(1):29-34.
9. Balagula Y, Rosen ST, Lacouture ME. The emergence of supportive oncodermatology: The study of dermatologic adverse events to cancer therapies. *J Am Acad Dermatol* 2011;65(3):624-35.
10. Lorusso D, Di Stefano A, Carone V, Fagotti A, Pisconti S, Scambia G. Pegylated liposomal doxorubicin-related palmar-plantar erythrodysesthesia ('hand-foot' syndrome). *Ann Oncol: ESMO* 2007;18(7):1159-64.
11. von Moos R et al. Pegylated liposomal doxorubicin-associated hand-foot syndrome: Recommendations of an international panel of experts. *Eur J Cancer* 2008;44(6):781-90.
12. Chen M et al. The contribution of keratinocytes in capecitabine-stimulated hand-foot-syndrome. *Environ Toxicol Pharmacol* 2017;49:81-8.
13. Yang J et al. The role of the ATM/Chk/P53 pathway in mediating DNA damage in hand-foot syndrome induced by PLD. *Toxicol Lett* 2017;265:131-9.

14. Lou Y et al. Possible pathways of capecitabine-induced hand-foot syndrome. *Chem Res Toxicol* 2016; 29(10):1591-601.
15. Zhang RX et al. Celecoxib can prevent capecitabine-related hand-foot syndrome in stage II and III colorectal cancer patients: Result of a single-center, prospective randomized phase III trial. *Ann Oncol: ESMO* 2012;23(5):1348-53.
16. Nikolaou V, Syrigos K, Saif MW. Incidence and implications of chemotherapy related hand-foot syndrome. *Expert Opin Drug Saf* 2016;15(12):1625-33.
17. Sibaud V, Meyer N, Lamant L, Vigarios E, Mazieres J, Delord JP. Dermatologic complications of anti-PD-1/PD-L1 immune checkpoint antibodies. *Curr Opin Oncol* 2016;28(4):254-63.
18. Syrigou E et al. Hypersensitivity reactions to docetaxel: Retrospective evaluation and development of a desensitization protocol. *Int Arch Allergy Immunol* 2011;156(3):320-4.
19. Aoyama T et al. Is there any predictor for hypersensitivity reactions in gynecologic cancer patients treated with paclitaxel-based therapy? *Cancer Chemother Pharmacol* 2017;80(1):65-9.
20. Gelmon K. The taxoids: Paclitaxel and docetaxel. *Lancet* 1994;344(8932):1267-72.
21. Park HJ et al. A new practical desensitization protocol for oxaliplatin-induced immediate hypersensitivity reactions: A necessary and useful approach. *J Investig Allergol Clin Immunol* 2016;26(3):168-76.
22. Langer SW. Extravasation of chemotherapy. *Curr Oncol Rep* 2010;12(4):242-6.
23. Kyllo R, Anadkat M. Dermatologic adverse events to chemotherapeutic agents, Part 1: Cytotoxic agents, epidermal growth factor inhibitors, multikinase inhibitors, and proteasome inhibitors. *Semin Cutan Med Surg* 2014;33(1):28-39.
24. Jain V, Bhandary S, Prasad GN, Shenoi SD. Serpentine supravenous streaks induced by 5-fluorouracil. *J Am Acad Dermatol* 2005;53(3):529-30.
25. Teresi ME, Murry DJ, Cornelius AS. Ifosfamide-induced hyperpigmentation. *Cancer* 1993;71(9):2873-5.
26. Chittari K, Tagboto S, Tan BB. Cyclophosphamide-induced nail discoloration and skin hyperpigmentation: A rare presentation. *Clin Exp Dermatol* 2009;34(3):405-6.
27. Abess A, Keel DM, Graham BS. Flagellate hyperpigmentation following intralesional bleomycin treatment of verruca plantaris. *Arch Dermatol* 2003;139(3):337-9.
28. Vuerstaek JD, Frank J, Poblete-Gutierrez P. Bleomycin-induced flagellate dermatitis. *Int J Dermatol* 2007(46 Suppl 3):3-5.
29. Huang V, Anadkat M. Dermatologic manifestations of cytotoxic therapy. *Dermatol Ther* 2011;24(4):401-10.
30. Suvirya S, Agrawal A, Parihar A. 5-Fluorouracil-induced bilateral persistent serpentine supravenous hyperpigmented eruption, bilateral mottling of palms and diffuse hyperpigmentation of soles. *BMJ Case Reports* 2014;2014.
31. Kyllo RL, Anadkat MJ. Dermatologic adverse events to chemotherapeutic agents, part 1: Cytotoxics, epidermal growth factor receptors, multikinase inhibitors, and proteasome inhibitors. *Semin Cutan Med Surg* 2014;33(1):28-39.
32. Capriotti K et al. The risk of nail changes with taxane chemotherapy: A systematic review of the literature and meta-analysis. *Br J Dermatol* 2015;173(3):842-5.
33. Trueb RM. Chemotherapy-induced hair loss. *Skin Therapy Lett* 2010;15(7):5-7.
34. Tallon B, Blanchard E, Goldberg LJ. Permanent chemotherapy-induced alopecia: Case report and review of the literature. *J Am Acad Dermatol* 2010;63(2):333-6.
35. Lindner J et al. Hair shaft abnormalities after chemotherapy and tamoxifen therapy in patients with

breast cancer evaluated by optical coherence tomography. *Br J Dermatol* 2012;167(6):1272-8.
36. Nangia J et al. Effect of a scalp cooling device on alopecia in women undergoing chemotherapy for breast cancer: The SCALP randomized clinical trial. *JAMA* 2017;317(6):596-605.
37. Trueb RM. Chemotherapy-induced anagen effluvium: Diffuse or patterned? *Dermatology* 2007;215(1):1-2.
38. Fonia A, Cota C, Setterfield JF, Goldberg LJ, Fenton DA, Stefanato CM. Permanent alopecia in patients with breast cancer after taxane chemotherapy and adjuvant hormonal therapy: Clinicopathologic findings in a cohort of 10 patients. *J Am Acad Dermatol* 2017;76(5):948-57.
39. Kluger N et al. Permanent scalp alopecia related to breast cancer chemotherapy by sequential fluorouracil/epirubicin/cyclophosphamide (FEC) and docetaxel: A prospective study of 20 patients. *Ann Oncol: ESMO* 2012;23(11):2879-84.
40. Miteva M, Misciali C, Fanti PA, Vincenzi C, Romanelli P, Tosti A. Permanent alopecia after systemic chemotherapy: A clinicopathological study of 10 cases. *Am J Dermatopathol* 2011;33(4):345-50.
41. Asz-Sigall D, Gonzalez-de-Cossio-Hernandez AC, Rodriguez-Lobato E, Ortega-Springall MF, Vega-Memije ME, Arenas Guzman R. Differential diagnosis of female-pattern hair loss. *Skin Appendage Disord* 2016;2(1-2):18-21.
42. Palamaras I, Misciali C, Vincenzi C, Robles WS, Tosti A. Permanent chemotherapy-induced alopecia: A review. *J Am Acad Dermatol* 2011;64(3):604-6.
43. Prevezas C, Matard B, Pinquier L, Reygagne P. Irreversible and severe alopecia following docetaxel or paclitaxel cytotoxic therapy for breast cancer. *Br J Dermatol* 2009;160(4):883-5.
44. Burris HA, 3rd, Hurtig J. Radiation recall with anticancer agents. *Oncologist* 2010;15(11):1227-37.
45. Sanborn RE, Sauer DA. Cutaneous reactions to chemotherapy: Commonly seen, less described, little understood. *Dermatol Clin* 2008;26(1):103-19, ix.
46. Wyatt AJ, Leonard GD, Sachs DL. Cutaneous reactions to chemotherapy and their management. *Am J Clin Dermatol* 2006;7(1):45-63.
47. Korman AM, Tyler KH, Kaffenberger BH. Radiation recall dermatitis associated with nivolumab for metastatic malignant melanoma. *Int J Dermatol* 2017;56(4):e75-7.
48. Belum VR, Fontanilla Patel H, Lacouture ME, Rodeck U. Skin toxicity of targeted cancer agents: Mechanisms and intervention. *Future Oncol* 2013;9(8):1161-70.
49. Tang N, Ratner D. Managing cutaneous side effects from targeted molecular inhibitors for melanoma and nonmelanoma skin cancer. *Dermatol Surg* 2016;42(Suppl 1):S40-8.
50. Belum VR, Washington C, Pratilas CA, Sibaud V, Boralevi F, Lacouture ME. Dermatologic adverse events in pediatric patients receiving targeted anticancer therapies: A pooled analysis. *Pediatr Blood Cancer* 2015;62(5):798-806.
51. Lacouture ME, Ciccolini K, Kloos RT, Agulnik M. Overview and management of dermatologic events associated with targeted therapies for medullary thyroid cancer. *Thyroid* 2014;24(9):1329-40.
52. Lacouture ME et al. Clinical practice guidelines for the prevention and treatment of EGFR inhibitor-associated dermatologic toxicities. *Support Care Cancer* 2011;19(8):1079-95.
53. Belum VR, Fischer A, Choi JN, Lacouture ME. Dermatological adverse events from BRAF inhibitors: A growing problem. *Curr Oncol Rep* 2013;15(3):249-59.
54. Tischer B, Huber R, Kraemer M, Lacouture ME. Dermatologic events from EGFR inhibitors: The issue of the missing patient voice. *Support Care Cancer* 2017;25(2):651-60.
55. Lacouture ME et al. A proposed EGFR inhibitor dermatologic adverse event-specific grading scale

from the MASCC skin toxicity study group. *Support Care Cancer* 2010;18(4):509-22.
56. Hofheinz RD et al. Recommendations for the prophylactic management of skin reactions induced by epidermal growth factor receptor inhibitors in patients with solid tumors. *Oncologist* 2016;21(12):1483-91.
57. Hsiao YW, Lin YC, Hui RC, Yang CH. Fulminant acneiform eruptions after administration of dovitinib in a patient with renal cell carcinoma. *J Clin Oncol* 2011;29(12):e340-1.
58. Drilon A et al. Beyond the dose-limiting toxicity period: Dermatologic adverse events of patients on phase 1 trials of the cancer therapeutics evaluation program. *Cancer* 2016;122(8):1228-37.
59. Clabbers JMK et al. Xerosis and pruritus as major EGFRI-associated adverse events. *Support Care Cancer* 2016;24(2):513-21.
60. Liu HB et al. Skin rash could predict the response to EGFR tyrosine kinase inhibitor and the prognosis for patients with non-small cell lung cancer: A systematic review and meta-analysis. *PLoS One* 2013;8(1):e55128.
61. Lacouture ME et al. Skin toxicity evaluation protocol with panitumumab (STEPP), a phase II, open-label, randomized trial evaluating the impact of a pre-emptive skin treatment regimen on skin toxicities and quality of life in patients with metastatic colorectal cancer. *J Clin Oncol* 2010;28(8):1351-7.
62. Dai J, Belum VR, Wu S, Sibaud V, Lacouture ME. Pigmentary changes in patients treated with targeted anticancer agents: A systematic review and meta-analysis. *J Am Acad Dermatol* 2017;77(5):902-10. e2.
63. Gandhi M, Brieva JC, Lacouture ME. Dermatologic infections in cancer patients. *Cancer Treat Res* 2014;161:299-317.
64. Macdonald JB, Macdonald B, Golitz LE, LoRusso P, Sekulic A. Cutaneous adverse effects of targeted therapies: Part II: Inhibitors of intracellular molecular signaling pathways. *J Am Acad Dermatol* 2015;72(2):221-36, quiz 37-8.
65. Lacouture ME et al. Evolving strategies for the management of hand-foot skin reaction associated with the multitargeted kinase inhibitors sorafenib and sunitinib. *Oncologist* 2008;13(9):1001-11.
66. Valentine J et al. Incidence and risk of xerosis with targeted anticancer therapies. *J Am Acad Dermatol* 2015;72(4):656-67.
67. Ensslin CJ, Rosen AC, Wu S, Lacouture ME. Pruritus in patients treated with targeted cancer therapies: Systematic review and meta-analysis. *J Am Acad Dermatol* 2013;69(5):708-20.
68. Gomez P, Lacouture ME. Clinical presentation and management of hand-foot skin reaction associated with sorafenib in combination with cytotoxic chemotherapy: Experience in breast cancer. *Oncologist* 2011;16(11):1508-19.
69. Lacouture ME, Reilly LM, Gerami P, Guitart J. Hand foot skin reaction in cancer patients treated with the multikinase inhibitors sorafenib and sunitinib. *Ann Oncol: ESMO* 2008;19(11):1955-61.
70. Lacouture ME et al. Dermatologic adverse events associated with afatinib: An oral ErbB family blocker. *Expert Rev Anticancer Ther* 2013;13(6):721-8.
71. Yeh CN et al. Fas/Fas ligand mediates keratinocyte death in sunitinib-induced hand-foot skin reaction. *J Invest Dermatol* 2014;134(11):2768-75.
72. Belum VR, Wu S, Lacouture ME. Risk of hand-foot skin reaction with the novel multikinase inhibitor regorafenib: A meta-analysis. *Investig New Drugs* 2013;31(4):1078-86.
73. Fischer A, Wu S, Ho AL, Lacouture ME. The risk of hand-foot skin reaction to axitinib, a novel VEGF inhibitor: A systematic review of literature and meta-analysis. *Investig New Drugs* 2013;31(3):787-97.

74. McLellan B, Ciardiello F, Lacouture ME, Segaert S, Van Cutsem E. Regorafenib-associated hand-foot skin reaction: Practical advice on diagnosis, prevention, and management. *Ann Oncol*: ESMO 2015;26(10):2017-26.
75. Balagula Y, Wu S, Su X, Feldman DR, Lacouture ME. The risk of hand foot skin reaction to pazopanib, a novel multikinase inhibitor: A systematic review of literature and meta-analysis. *Investig New Drugs* 2012;30(4):1773-81.
76. Carlos G et al. Cutaneous toxic effects of BRAF inhibitors alone and in combination with MEK inhibitors for metastatic melanoma. *JAMA Dermatol* 2015;151(10):1103-9.
77. Choi JN. Dermatologic adverse events to chemotherapeutic agents, Part 2: BRAF inhibitors, MEK inhibitors, and ipilimumab. *Semin Cutan Med Surg* 2014;33(1):40-8.
78. Belum VR, Cercek A, Sanz-Motilva V, Lacouture ME. Dermatologic adverse events to targeted therapies in lower GI cancers: Clinical presentation and management. *Curr Treat Options Oncol* 2013;14(3):389-404.
79. Pugliese SB, Neal JW, Kwong BY. Management of dermatologic complications of lung cancer therapies. *Curr Treat Options Oncol* 2015;16(10):50.
80. Chandrakumar SF, Yeung J. Cutaneous adverse events during vemurafenib therapy. *J Cutan Med Surg* 2014;18(4):223-8.
81. Balagula Y, Barth Huston K, Busam KJ, Lacouture ME, Chapman PB, Myskowski PL. Dermatologic side effects associated with the MEK 1/2 inhibitor selumetinib (AZD6244, ARRY-142886). *Investig New Drugs* 2011;29(5):1114-21.
82. Dreno B et al. Incidence, course, and management of toxicities associated with cobimetinib in combination with vemurafenib in the coBRIM study. *Ann Oncol*: ESMO 2017;28(5):1137-44.
83. Keating GM. Cobimetinib plus vemurafenib: A review in BRAF (V600) mutation-positive unresectable or metastatic melanoma. *Drugs* 2016;76(5):605-15.
84. Lacouture ME et al. Characterization and management of hedgehog pathway inhibitor-related adverse events in patients with advanced basal cell carcinoma. *Oncologist* 2016;21(10):1218-29.
85. Kwong B, Danial C, Liu A, Chun KA, Chang AL. Reversible cutaneous side effects of vismodegib treatment. *Cutis* 2017;99(3):19-20.
86. LoRusso PM et al. Phase I trial of hedgehog pathway inhibitor vismodegib (GDC-0449) in patients with refractory, locally advanced or metastatic solid tumors. *Clin Cancer Res* 2011;17(8):2502-11.
87. Sekulic A et al. Long-term safety and efficacy of vismodegib in patients with advanced basal cell carcinoma: final update of the pivotal ERIVANCE BCC study. *BMC Cancer* 2017;17(1):332.
88. Aasi S et al. New onset of keratoacanthomas after vismodegib treatment for locally advanced basal cell carcinomas: A report of 2 cases. *JAMA Dermatol* 2013;149(2):242-3.
89. Sekulic A et al. Efficacy and safety of vismodegib in advanced basal-cell carcinoma. *N Engl J Med* 2012;366(23):2171-9.
90. U.S. Food and Drug Administration. Vismodegib. January 2012. https://www.accessdata.fda.gov/drugsatfda_docs/label/2012/203388lbl.pdf. Accessed June 26,2017.
91. European Medicines Agency. European Public Assessment Report: Erivedge. October 2016. http://www.ema.europa.eu/docs/en_GB/document_library/EPAR_-_Summary_for_the_public/human/002602/WC500146821.pdf.
92. Weber JS, Yang JC, Atkins MB, Disis ML. Toxicities of immunotherapy for the practitioner. *J Clin Oncol* 2015;33(18):2092-9.
93. Michot JM et al. Immune-related adverse events with immune checkpoint blockade: A comprehensive review. *Eur J Cancer* 2016;54:139-48.

94. Wolchok JD et al. Ipilimumab monotherapy in patients with pretreated advanced melanoma: A randomised, double-blind, multicentre, phase 2, dose-ranging study. *Lancet Oncol* 2010;11(2):155-64.
95. Postow MA, Sidlow R, Hellmann MD. Immune-related adverse events associated with immune checkpoint blockade. *N Engl J Med* 2018;378(2):158-68.
96. Larsabal M et al. Vitiligo-like lesions occurring in patients receiving anti-programmed cell death-1 therapies are clinically and biologically distinct from vitiligo. *J Am Acad Dermatol* 2017;76(5):863-70.
97. Belum VR et al. Characterisation and management of dermatologic adverse events to agents targeting the PD-1 receptor. *Eur J Cancer* 2016;60:12-25.
98. Robert C et al. Pembrolizumab versus ipilimumab in advanced melanoma. *N Engl J Med* 2015;372(26):2521-32.
99. Naidoo J et al. Autoimmune bullous skin disorders with immune checkpoint inhibitors targeting PD-1 and PD-L1. *Cancer Immunol Res* 2016;4(5):383-9.
100. Damsky W, King BA. JAK inhibitors in dermatology: The promise of a new drug class. *J Am Acad Dermatol* 2017;76(4):736-44.
101. Shreberk-Hassidim R, Ramot Y, Zlotogorski A. Janus kinase inhibitors in dermatology: A systematic review. *J Am Acad Dermatol* 2017;76(4):745-53. e19.
102. Sibaud V et al. Oral lichenoid reactions associated with anti-PD-1/PD-L1 therapies: Clinicopathological findings. *J Eur Acad Dermatol Venereol* 2017;31(10):e464-9.
103. Weber JS, Dummer R, de Pril V, Lebbe C, Hodi FS, MDX010-20 Investigators. Patterns of onset and resolution of immune-related adverse events of special interest with ipilimumab: Detailed safety analysis from a phase 3 trial in patients with advanced melanoma. *Cancer* 2013;119(9):1675-82.
104. Curry JL et al. Diverse types of dermatologic toxicities from immune checkpoint blockade therapy. *J Cutan Pathol* 2017;44(2):158-76.
105. Freeman-Keller M, Kim Y, Cronin H, Richards A, Gibney G, Weber JS. Nivolumab in resected and unresectable metastatic melanoma: Characteristics of immune-related adverse events and association with outcomes. *Clin Cancer Res* 2016;22(4):886-94.
106. Goldinger SM et al. Cytotoxic cutaneous adverse drug reactions during anti-PD-1 therapy. *Clin Cancer Res* 2016;22(16):4023-9.
107. Weber JS, Kahler KC, Hauschild A. Management of immune-related adverse events and kinetics of response with ipilimumab. *J Clin Oncol* 2012;30(21):2691-7.
108. Jour G et al. Autoimmune dermatologic toxicities from immune checkpoint blockade with anti-PD-1 antibody therapy: A report on bullous skin eruptions. *J Cutan Pathol* 2016;43(8):688-96.
109. Nayar N, Briscoe K, Fernandez Penas P. Toxic epidermal necrolysis-like reaction with severe satellite cell necrosis associated with nivolumab in a patient with ipilimumab refractory metastatic melanoma. *J Immunother* 2016;39(3):149-52.
110. Johnson DB et al. Severe cutaneous and neurologic toxicity in melanoma patients during vemurafenib administration following anti-PD-1 therapy. *Cancer Immunol Res* 2013;1(6):373-7.
111. Voskens CJ et al. The price of tumor control: An analysis of rare side effects of anti-CTLA-4 therapy in metastatic melanoma from the ipilimumab network. *PLoS One* 2013;8(1):e53745.
112. Wong RK et al. Clinical practice guidelines for the prevention and treatment of acute and late radiation reactions from the MASCC skin toxicity study group. *Support Care Cancer* 2013;21(10):2933-48.
113. Shaitelman SF et al. Acute and short-term toxic effects of conventionally fractionated vs hypofractionated whole-breast irradiation: A randomized clinical trial. *JAMA Oncol* 2015;1(7):

931-41.
114. Hymes SR, Alousi AM, Cowen EW. Graft-versus-host disease: Part I. Pathogenesis and clinical manifestations of graft-versus-host disease. *J Am Acad Dermatol* 2012;66(4):515. e1-18, quiz 33-4.
115. Villarreal CD, Alanis JC, Perez JC, Candiani JO. Cutaneous graft-versus-host disease after hematopoietic stem cell transplant: A review. *Anais Brasileiros de Dermatologia* 2016;91(3):336-43.

第二章

痤疮样皮疹

加布里埃拉·法布罗奇尼(Gabriella Fabbrocini),玛丽亚·康塞塔·罗曼诺(Maria Concetta Romano),萨拉·卡奇亚普奥蒂(Sara Cacciapuoti),路易吉娅·帕纳列洛(Luigia Panariello)

金尚霖 译

一 背景

痤疮样皮疹(acneiform eruption)定义为类似于寻常痤疮的皮肤病。皮损可以是丘疹脓疱性、结节状或囊性。痤疮样皮疹通常缺乏粉刺,而寻常痤疮通常具有粉刺。

本章重点介绍表皮生长因子受体(EGFR)抑制剂诱导的痤疮样皮疹,这是肿瘤患者在使用这些新药治疗过程中最常见的皮肤不良反应之一。常见导致痤疮样皮疹的 EFGR 抑制剂及其作用机制见表 2-1。

表 2-1 常见导致痤疮样皮疹的 EGFR 抑制剂及其作用机制

药物分子结构	药物名称	作用机制
单克隆抗体	西妥昔单抗(爱必妥®) 帕尼单抗(维克替比®) 耐昔妥珠单抗	细胞外结合 EGFR,抑制其活化
小分子	吉非替尼(易瑞沙®) 厄洛替尼(特罗凯®) 阿法替尼(吉泰瑞®) 达克替尼 拉帕替尼(泰立沙®) 奥希替尼(泰瑞沙®)	抑制 EGFR 细胞内酪氨酸激酶结构域,阻止下游信号级联的活化

考虑到 EGFR 的作用机制以及在人类皮肤中的分布多效性,抗体和酪氨酸激酶抑制剂均能产生痤疮样皮疹,且频率高达 80%,也就不足为奇了。此类药疹是 EGFR 抑制剂治疗过程中最常见的皮肤不良事件。据报道,它发生于 50%~100%的患者中[1-4]。

痤疮样皮疹是一种剂量依赖的皮肤药物反应,常发生在治疗最初的 1~2 周,并于 3~4 周达到高峰。典型皮疹是皮脂腺丰富区域出现炎性丘疹、脓疱,并伴瘙痒。EGFR 抑制剂治疗后出现痤疮样皮疹,往往预示着良好的治疗反应[5]。该病可以影响患者的生活质量,有时会导致抗肿瘤治疗的停止。

二 发病机制

这些 EGFR 抑制剂同时抑制肿瘤细胞和正常表皮细胞中的 EGFR。角质形成细胞中的 EGFR 被抑制后会诱导细胞凋亡、阻止细胞生长、减少细胞迁移,并增加细胞黏附和细胞分化(图 2-1)。细胞生长停滞、角质形成细胞迁移以及炎症反应,导致皮肤干燥和痤疮样疹。

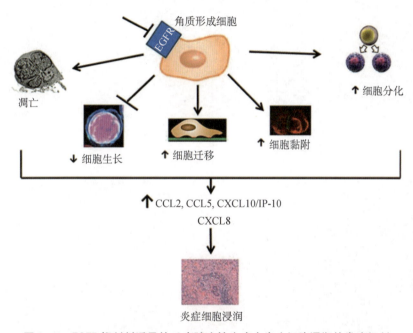

图 2-1　EGFR 抑制剂诱导的丘疹脓疱性皮疹中炎症细胞浸润的发病机制

三 临床表现

痤疮样皮疹患者表现出痤疮样病变,如丘疹和脓疱。皮疹消退后,通常无后遗症。痤疮样皮疹最常见的并发症是脓疱化。当皮疹突然加重(皮疹更加多形性、有典型的蜂蜜色痂),应怀疑细菌性脓疱。脓疱化最常见的细菌是金黄色葡萄球菌,尤其是鼻腔带菌者和躯干受累的患者(图 2-2~图 2-6)[6]。

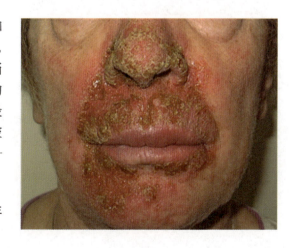

图 2-2　使用帕尼单抗治疗结直肠癌的患者发生面部痤疮样皮疹,2 级

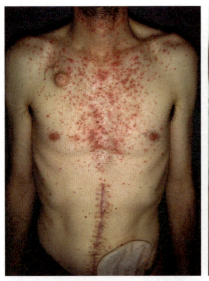

图2-3 使用帕尼单抗+氟尿嘧啶+伊立替康的患者发生躯干痤疮样皮疹,2级

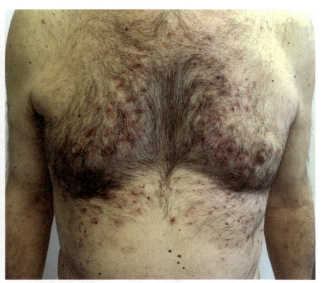

图2-4 使用阿法替尼的患者发生继发性感染

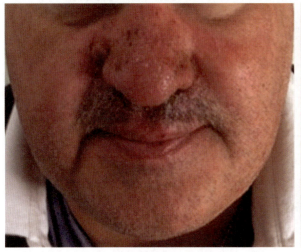

图2-5 使用厄洛替尼的患者发生痤疮样皮疹,1级

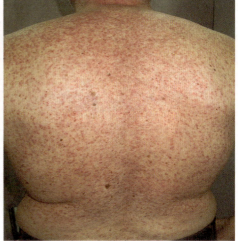

图2-6 使用吉非替尼的患者发生痤疮样皮疹,2级

四 组织学

受累区域的活检标本可见角质层更薄、更致密,偶见局灶角化不全,正常的网篮状外观消失,伴有轻度的颗粒层减少,有明显的角栓形成和毛囊漏斗部扩张[7]。

五 治疗

已提出的各种治疗策略和建议,是基于个例报道、临床经验、专家共识及小样本量的随机试验[1,8]。这可能是因为很难招募到大量有明确病变特点的患者开展临床试验。

治疗应个体化,取决于皮疹的严重程度(表2-2)[9-11]。

表2-2 按等级治疗EGFR抑制剂引起的毛囊炎

	治疗措施	1级	2级	3~4级
药物治疗	口服抗生素(多西环素 100~200 mg/d)、抗组胺药	除了支持性预防措施外,口服四环素类药物(米诺环素 100 mg/d,赖甲环素 300 mg/d 或者多西环素 100 mg/d)	外用类固醇激素,如2.5%氢化可的松乳膏	口服大剂量四环素类药物(米诺环素 100 mg/d、赖甲环素 300 mg/d 或多西环素 100 mg/d,均连续 2 d) 除了2级治疗外,口服类固醇激素(泼尼松 0.5 mg/kg,连续 5 d) 经治疗 2~4 周后,若毒性反应仍无减轻,需考虑减少药物剂量或停止 EGFR 抑制剂治疗 怀疑二重感染:细菌和/或病毒拭子检查
支持性护肤产品	润肤剂和保湿霜 pH值5.5、不含香精的洁肤剂 防光保护 治疗性化妆	同样的皮肤护理产品	同样的皮肤护理产品	同样的皮肤护理产品

作为预防性治疗,可口服具有抗炎作用的抗生素(如多西环素 100~200 mg/d)或抗组胺药物,并联合外用类固醇激素。考虑到刺激性不良反应,许多治疗痤疮的药物应避免使用,如过氧化苯甲酰和维A酸类药物。患者应避免直接光照或日光浴、炎热或湿热的环境。油腻的霜剂,如凡士林具有高效润肤作用,但另一方面,其阻塞的特点容易产生毛囊炎。

当皮疹达到2级时,建议外用类固醇激素(2.5%氢化可的松乳膏)[12]。根据我们的经验和既往研究,患者外用克林霉素或红霉素亦有效。若患者自觉瘙痒,可外用薄荷乳膏或口服某种抗组胺药物。另外,可加服四环素类药物以达到抗炎作用(如米诺环素 100 mg/d、赖甲环素 300 mg/d 或多西环素 100 mg/d)[12,13]。亦有建议低剂量异维A酸治疗[12]。

当痤疮样皮疹严重(3级或4级)时,除前述治疗外,应加服大剂量四环素类药物(米诺环素 100 mg/d、赖甲环素 300 mg/d 或多西环素 100 mg/d,均连续 2 d)。当急性期消退,可减少治疗剂量。怀疑二重感染时,应给予细菌和/或病毒检查(如拭子),必要时适当口服或静脉使用抗生素。亦可加用口服类固醇激素(泼尼松 0.5 mg/kg,连续 5 d)[12]。

3级和4级皮疹经过2~4周治疗后,若毒性反应仍无减轻,则可考虑减少药物剂量或中断EGFR抑制剂治疗。

除了药物治疗外,有必要向所有接受EGFR抑制剂治疗的患者推荐特定的皮肤美容方案,因为利用美容管理可调整细胞更替时间、修复受损的角质层屏障。根据我们的经验,在抗肿瘤治疗初始,就应当积极采取皮肤美容方案,目的是通过产品中的一些物质模仿EGFR的作用(植物脂肪或化学脂肪与抗氧化分子结合),使皮肤对EGFR抑制剂诱导的过程不再易感。

此外,采取预防措施恢复皮肤屏障的完整性和水平衡,对治疗痤疮样皮疹相关干燥症至关重要,因为它们支持皮肤与美容产品之间产生生化亲和力。这些措施如下:使用不含水的配方(油剂、软膏、霜剂),选择植物脂肪而不是矿物脂肪。患者皮肤的日常护理要注重清洁、保湿和修复,推荐使用无酒精的油-软膏配方。

春季和夏季应使用广谱防晒霜。

为了减少1级和2级皮疹对生活质量的影响,可以使用特定的非封闭性化妆品,这类产品所有患者通常都能很好耐受的。建议使用富含脂肪酸和神经酰胺的化妆品配方以保护皮肤角质层屏障。

皮肤科医师应当注意是否存在二重感染的体征,尤其是金黄色葡萄球菌,但也可能是真菌或病毒感染。如果存疑,应进行皮肤拭子检查。

有趣的是,使用 EGFR 抑制剂治疗的患者,若出现细菌、真菌或病毒二重感染的丘疹脓疱性皮疹,至少有 30% 存在鼻咽腔内金黄色葡萄球菌定植;相比之下,在未发生皮肤感染的患者中,仅有 2.2% 出现定植。因此,对于存在丘疹脓疱性皮疹的患者,建议在鼻腔内使用莫匹罗星软膏,预防继发感染的风险。

六 预防

对于使用 EGFR 抑制剂治疗的患者,预防性治疗很关键,以预防和减少皮肤反应的严重度。抗肿瘤治疗开始、未出现不良反应之前,护理好患者,是避免皮疹发生或辅助治疗的正确选择。

在 EGFR 抑制剂治疗开始前,患者应被告知这种特定的皮肤不良事件。应建议患者尽可能地减少光暴露,因为皮疹可能在曝光部位更加严重。患者应避免使用碱性肥皂以及含酒精成分的香水或洗剂。患者日常的皮肤护理与"治疗"中描述相同。

一些研究发现口服抗生素可作为预防性治疗,尤其是四环素类抗生素,如多西环素(100～200 mg/d)或米诺环素 100 mg/d[12]。这类抗生素具有抗炎和组织保护的作用。对于肾功能不全的患者,使用多西环素是安全的选项;而米诺环素适用于夏季或高 UV 指数的地区,因为其光敏性较低[14]。

应在 EGFR 抑制剂治疗开始的首日给予抗生素,因为使用首剂 EGFR 抑制剂后,最早在 2 d 后即可发生毒性反应。尽管如此,根据我们的经验,预防性治疗可以降低痤疮样皮疹的发生和等级,让皮肤科医生可以避免系统使用抗生素。系统使用抗生素应当仅在外用治疗出现抵抗或发生二重感染时才进行。

七 鉴别诊断

EGFR 抑制剂诱发的丘疹脓疱性皮疹可合并细菌感染,尤其是金黄色葡萄球菌感染。而细菌性毛囊炎可表现为类似的丘疹脓疱性皮疹,因此可能被误诊。罕见因没有及时应用抗生素治疗而导致血行感染,尤其是在有免疫抑制的患者中。

医生可通过以下两点区分丘疹脓疱性皮疹和细菌性毛囊炎：部位和发生时间[15]。发生在以下部位需怀疑二重感染：上下肢、下腹部、臀部和腹股沟。EGFR 抑制剂治疗 12 周后出现的新发皮疹，无论发生在什么部位，都应怀疑细菌性二重感染。

八 结语

痤疮样皮疹是 EGFR 抑制剂最常见的皮肤不良事件。随着 EGFR 抑制剂应用的增加，诊断和处理其不良反应，确保患者对抗肿瘤治疗的依从和坚持，将变得非常重要。

丘疹脓疱性皮疹的发病机制及组织学改变还有待进一步研究，以推进更标准化的治疗策略和预防措施。

参 考 文 献

1. Chanprapaph K, Vachiramon V, Rattanakaemakorn P. Epidermal growth factor receptor inhibitors: A review of cutaneous adverse events and management. *Dermatol Res Pract* 2014;2014:734249.
2. Segaert S, Van Custem E. Clinical signs, pathophysiology and management of skin toxicity during therapy with epidermal growth factor receptor inhibitors. *Ann Oncol* 2005;16(9):1425-33.
3. Jacot W et al. Acneiform eruption induced by epidermal growth factor receptor inhibitors in patients with solid tumours. *Br J Dermatol* 2004;151:238-41.
4. Ha KD, Navid E, Wolverton ES. Drug induced acneiform eruptions. In: Zeichner JA, ed. *Acneiform Eruptions in Dermatology*. 1st ed. New York, NY: Springer-Verlag; 2014; pp. 389-404.
5. Journagan S, Obadiah J. An acneiform eruption due to erlotinib: Prognostic implications and management. *J Am Acad Dermatol* 2006;54:358-60.
6. Peuvrel L, Bachmeyer C, Reguiai Z, Bachet JB, André T, Bensadoun RJ et al. Semiology of skin toxicity associated with epidermal growth factor receptor (EGFR) inhibitors. *Support Care Cancer* 2012;20:909-21.
7. Vanhoefer U, Tewes M, Rojo F, Dirsch O, Schleucher N, Rosen O et al. Phase I study of the humanized antiepidermal growth factor receptor monoclonal antibody EMD72000 in patients with advanced solid tumors that express the epidermal growth factor receptor. *J Clin Oncol* 2004;22:175-84.
8. Liu S, Kurzrock R. Understanding toxicities of targeted agents: Implications for anti-tumor activity and management. *Semin Oncol* 2015 Dec;42(6):863-75.
9. Dreno B, Bensadoun RJ, Humbert P, Krutmann J, Luger T, Triller R et al. Algorithm for dermocosmetic use in the management of cutaneous side-effects associated with targeted therapy in oncology. *J Eur Acad Dermatol Venereol* 2013;27:1071-80.
10. Liu S, Kurzrock R. Understanding toxicities of targeted agents: Implications for anti-tumor activity and management. *Semin Oncol* 2015;42:863-75.
11. Hofheinz RD, Deplanque G, Komatsu Y, Kobayashi Y, Ocvirk J, Racca P et al. Recommendations for the prophylactic management of skin reactions induced by epidermal growth factor receptor inhibitors in patients with solid tumors. *Oncologist* 2016;21:1483-491.
12. Lacouture ME, Anadkat M, Jatoi A, Garawin T, Bohac C, Mitchell E. Dermatologic toxicity occurring during anti-EGFR monoclonal inhibitor therapy in patients with metastatic colorectal

cancer: A systematic review. *Clin Colorectal Cancer* 2018;17(2):85-96.
13. Grande R, Narducci F, Bianchetti S, Mansueto G, Gemma D, Sperduti I et al. Pre-emptive skin toxicity treatment for anti-EGFR drugs: Evaluation of efficacy of skin moisturizers and lymecycline. A phase II study. *Support Care Cancer* 2013;21(6):1691-695.
14. Stulhofer Buzina D, Martinac I, Ledic DD, Ceovic R, Bilic I, Marinovic B. The most common cutaneous side effects of epidermal growth factor receptor inhibitors and their management. *Acta Dermatovenerol Croat* 2015;23:282-88.
15. Braden R, Anadkat M. EGFR inhibitor-induced skin reactions: Differentiating acneiform rash from superimposed bacterial infections. *Support Care Cancer* 2016;24:3943-950.

第三章

毛发疾病

阿泽尔·弗雷特斯·马丁内斯(Azael Freites-Martinez),加布里埃拉·法布罗奇尼(Gabriella Fabbrocini),马里奥·拉库蒂尔(Mario E. Lacouture),安东内拉·托斯蒂(Antonella Tosti)

盛友渔 韩中颖 张 波 译

一 概述

肿瘤患者最常见的毛发疾病是化疗所致脱发(CIA)[1]。然而,其他一些抗肿瘤疗法也可能与脱发及其他毛发病症相关,包括放疗、靶向治疗、免疫治疗、干细胞移植和内分泌治疗。此外,也可出现头发生长、色素和质地的改变,尽管在肿瘤患者中还没有被系统地报道。患儿和乳腺癌患者罹患持续性或永久性脱发的风险增加,其发生率分别高达14%[2]和30%[3]。持续性或永久性脱发的患者更容易由于情绪问题而损害情感功能,即自尊或自我形象受到负面影响[2]。

本章综述了肿瘤患者和幸存者由于抗肿瘤治疗导致的各类毛发疾病,并提供针对这些病症的适当处理方法。

二 传统抗肿瘤治疗引起的毛发病症

(一) 细胞毒性化疗

1. 化疗所致脱发

CIA通常在首次细胞毒性化疗后几天到几周内发生,表现为非瘢痕性、斑片状或弥漫性生长期脱发,主要发生于易摩擦部位,如头顶和颞枕区域,可能在2～3个月内进展至头发完全脱落。韩国的一项研究表明,化疗所致的生长期脱发并非均匀地影响头皮,男性后发际和女性前发际区域脱发较轻微[4]。除了脱发,还可见身体其他部位的毛发脱落。CIA的毛发镜检查示生长期脱发,包括黑点征、黄点征、感叹号样发,以及发干颜色和粗细的变化(图3-1)。虽然不同药物所致CIA的临床表现类似(表3-1),但越来越多的证据表明它们的分子生物学基础是不同的,受到个体易感性的影响[5]。

2. 化疗所致持续性脱发

化疗所致持续性脱发(pCIA)又称化疗后永久性脱发,是指化疗停止6个月后持续脱发,其发生率在乳腺癌幸存者中高达30%[3],在儿童癌症幸存者中高达14%[2]。pCIA主

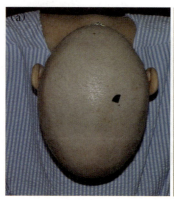
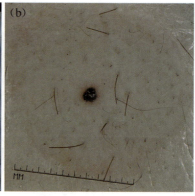

图 3-1 化疗所致脱发

(a)使用第一剂多西他赛 6 周后的临床表现；(b)毛发镜检查示：黑点征、黄点征和断发

表 3-1 常致可逆性或持续性脱发的抗肿瘤疗法

抗肿瘤疗法	明确或正在研究的肿瘤类型	可逆性脱发发生率	持续性脱发发生率
化疗			
环磷酰胺	乳腺癌、白血病、淋巴瘤、多发性骨髓瘤、神经母细胞瘤、视网膜母细胞瘤、卵巢癌	25%（低剂量），约100%（高剂量）	报道主要是以紫杉烷为基础的化疗（30%）
柔红霉素、多柔比星和伊达比星	急性髓系白血病、急性淋巴细胞白血病、甲状腺癌、乳腺癌、胃癌、肺癌、膀胱癌、淋巴瘤、神经母细胞瘤、肉瘤、肾母细胞瘤	约100%	
紫杉烷类（多西他赛、紫杉醇）	乳腺癌、胃癌、头颈癌、肺癌、前列腺癌	约100%	30%
依托泊苷	小细胞肺癌、睾丸癌	约55%	
伊立替康和拓扑替康	结直肠癌、小细胞肺癌、卵巢癌、宫颈癌	约50%	
放疗			
光子放疗（传统放疗）和质子放疗	原发性中枢神经系统肿瘤、脑转移、头颈癌	75%～100%	高剂量分割照射 43 Gy（光子放疗）的风险高达 50%
靶向治疗			
维莫德吉	基底细胞癌（局部晚期或不能切除）	62%	报道很少
索拉非尼	肝细胞癌、肾细胞癌、甲状腺癌	26%	
舒尼替尼和瑞格非尼	转移性肾细胞癌、胃肠道间质瘤	4%～6%	
维莫非尼和达拉非尼	黑素瘤（Ⅳ期）	19%～24%	

(续表)

抗肿瘤疗法	明确或正在研究的肿瘤类型	可逆性脱发发生率	持续性脱发发生率
免疫治疗			
细胞毒性T淋巴细胞相关蛋白4（CTLA-4）	黑素瘤（Ⅲ～Ⅳ期）	1%～2%	
程序性死亡［蛋白］-1（PD-1）和程序性死亡受体1（PD-L1）	黑素瘤（Ⅳ期）、肺癌、霍奇金淋巴瘤、尿路上皮癌	2%	
干细胞移植			
预处理化疗（白消安、拓扑替康、噻替哌、依托泊苷、环磷酰胺）	白血病	约100%	30%
移植物抗宿主病		20%	20%
内分泌治疗			
亮丙瑞林	乳腺癌、肝细胞癌、神经内分泌肿瘤	2%	约25%（乳腺癌幸存者中）
奥曲肽		6.7%	
芳香化酶抑制剂（阿那曲唑、来曲唑、依西美坦）	转移性雌激素受体阳性（ER+）乳腺癌	约25%	

要见于接受紫杉烷类药物为基础的化疗方案（紫杉醇和多西他赛）[6]以及其他化疗方案（如环磷酰胺、噻替哌和卡铂）治疗的乳腺癌幸存者，以及接受白消安（单独或与环磷酰胺联合）骨髓移植预处理方案[7]（见表3-1）和放疗的患儿。

pCIA有多种临床特征（表3-2），最常见的是弥漫性非瘢痕性脱发，伴有头发强度、质地、长度和颜色改变（图3-2）。雄激素敏感部位的头皮脱发常更严重，可能误诊为雄激素性秃发（图3-3）。pCIA也可累及腋毛、阴毛、睫毛和眉毛。如其他类型脱发，临床特征是非特异性的，需要完整的病史询问和全身检查以确定医源性或任何其他可能的脱发原因。毛发镜检查可以看到营养不良性和微小化的毛发（图3-4）。

表3-2 抗肿瘤治疗引起毛发病症的临床特征

抗肿瘤疗法	临床特征
化疗	(1) 脱发:非瘢痕性脱发,常于头皮易摩擦区域起病,主要是生长期脱发。通常在最后一个化疗周期6个月后完全恢复。通常会观察到身体其他部位的毛发脱落。毛发镜检查示非特异性,见黑点征、黄点征、感叹号样发,以及头发颜色和粗细变化 (2) 头发颜色和质地变化:颜色变深和变浅。直发可能变卷曲或波浪状,并且更细,通常在最后一个化疗周期后6个月恢复 (3) 多毛症:主要在面部 (4) 持续性化疗所致脱发:①有报道呈弥漫性头发稀疏,也有报道与雄激素性秃发相似的模式。变化主要是头发稀疏;②有报道呈瘢痕性脱发特征;③其他体毛也可受累及
放疗	(1) 脱发:非瘢痕性脱发;脱发区域形状与放疗区域相关。可见放射性皮炎。毛发镜检查示非特异性,包括黄点征、黑点征、短毳毛、毛周征和断发 (2) 头发颜色和质地改变:可见头发颜色变浅和变细 (3) 放疗所致持续性脱发:常见瘢痕性脱发特征,严重者伴皮肤萎缩、毛发稀疏。全脑照射联合细胞毒化疗导致弥漫性毛发稀疏
靶向治疗	(1) 脱发:严重毛囊炎症反应(如头皮糜烂脓疱性皮病、丛状毛囊炎)后出现非瘢痕和瘢痕性弥漫性脱发 (2) 多毛症和睫毛粗长症:多毛症和眼周多毛症常见于女性。睫毛和眉毛增多很常见,长而卷曲的睫毛可能影响视力(主要是EGFR抑制剂) (3) 头发颜色和质地改变:头发颜色改变,包括颜色变浅(VEGFR/PDGFR)和变深(EGFR抑制剂)
免疫治疗	(1) 脱发:弥漫性头发稀疏和斑秃 (2) 头发颜色改变:颜色变浅和变深
干细胞移植	(1) 脱发:类似于化疗所致的瘢痕性脱发,与预处理化疗有关;斑秃伴发移植物抗宿主病 (2) 头发颜色和质地改变:头发颜色变浅和稀疏 (3) 持续性毛发改变:可见具有瘢痕特征的弥漫性脱发(类似于化疗所致持续性脱发)
维莫德吉	(1) 脱发:与化疗类似 (2) 持续性毛发改变:持续性脱发罕有报道(类似化疗所致持续性脱发)
内分泌治疗	(1) 脱发:模式型脱发,类似雄激素性秃发 (2) 多毛症:可见多毛症

注:EGFR,表皮生长因子受体;VEGFR,血管内皮生长因子受体;PDGFR,血小板衍生生长因子受体。

抗肿瘤治疗引起的永久性或持续性脱发的组织病理学特征是在无纤维化的情况下毛囊总数严重减少。pCIA的其他特征包括毛囊微小化和休止期毛囊数量增加[8],以及网状真皮和皮下组织中纤维束(中柱)数量增加[9,10]。pCIA的其他非典型组织病理学特征包括瘢痕性脱发、同心性纤维化和毛囊周围散在的淋巴样细胞浸润[10](见图3-4)。

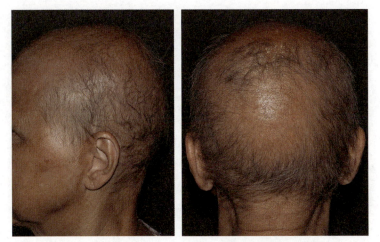

图 3-2 化疗所致持续性脱发 1

弥漫性头发稀疏和变色。最后一个周期紫杉醇化疗 3 年后的临床表现。

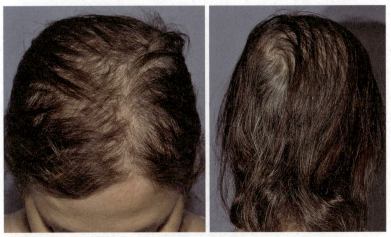

图 3-3 化疗所致持续性脱发 2

与雄激素性秃发类似。最后一个周期紫杉醇化疗 18 个月后的临床表现。

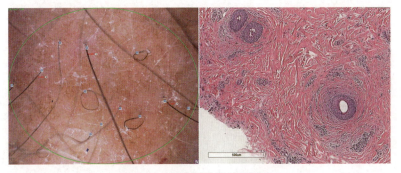

图 3-4 化疗所致持续性脱发 3

毛发镜检查示单根毳毛和营养不良发的毛囊单位。组织病理学检查（HE，500 μm）示毛囊总数减少，毛囊周围轻度淋巴细胞性炎症和纤维化。

(二) 放疗

1. 放疗所致脱发

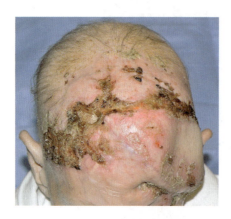

图 3-5 放疗引起脱发

光子放疗(传统放疗)后脱发伴头皮溃疡和结痂。

放疗所致脱发(radiotherapy-induced alopecia, RIA)的特征是生长期脱发,随后因毛囊过早进入退行期而出现休止期脱发。通常在第一次照射后 1~3 周观察到局限于放疗区域的几何形状脱发斑片(见表 3-2),并且通常在放疗 2~4 个月后头发完全再生。高达 45% 的病例中可见其他皮肤不良事件,包括红斑、放射性皮炎和溃疡(图 3-5),在急性期需要额外关注[11]。在 60% 的 RIA 中,毛发镜检查主要见黄点征和黑点征,其次是短毳毛、毛周征和断发[12]。

2. 放疗所致持续性脱发

放疗所致持续性脱发(persistent radiotherapy-induced alopecia, pRIA)界定为停止放疗 6 个月后头发尚未完全再生。这通常与头皮的高剂量放疗有关(光子放疗通常 > 30 Gy,质子放疗 > 21 Gy)。pRIA 的临床表现包括界限分明的、通常无症状的脱发和局限于放疗区域的皮肤萎缩(图 3-6)。如果照射剂量较低,休止期毛囊通常不会受到影响,因此脱发可呈不完全性[13]。

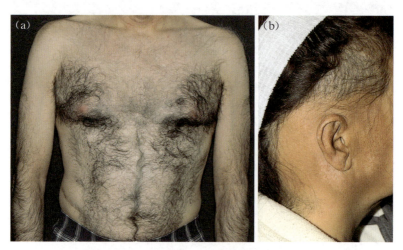

图 3-6 放疗所致持续性脱发和头发改变

(a)斗篷野放疗后躯干脱毛和毛发变白;(b)颞部头皮照射后持续性脱发。

(三) 内分泌治疗

内分泌治疗所致脱发(endocrine therapy-induced alopecia, EIA)的荟萃分析显示,所

有级别脱发的总发生率为 4.4%,重度脱发(脱发面积＞50%头皮面积)的发生率为 1.2%,接受他莫昔芬治疗的患者脱发发病率最高(所有级别总发生率为 25.4%)[14]。脱发的平均时间为 17 个月[15,16]。这些患者常表现为前额发际线后移和顶部稀疏,类似于雄激素性秃发的典型模式(图 3-7)。EIA 患者的毛发镜检查示雄激素性秃发特征(图 3-8)。有报道接受内分泌治疗(endocrine therapy, ET)的乳腺癌患者发生医源性多毛症[17]。

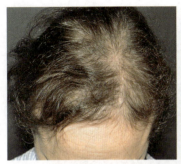
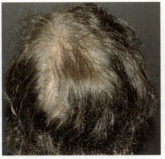

图 3-7 内分泌治疗所致脱发 1
类似于雄激素性秃发的模式。阿那曲唑治疗 12 个月后的临床表现。

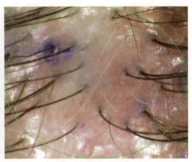

图 3-8 内分泌治疗所致脱发 2
头皮冠状区的毛发镜检查显示每个毛囊单位有一根头发和多根毳毛。

对于在细胞毒性化疗后接受内分泌治疗的患者,必须获得完整的病史以确定脱发是由于内分泌治疗(EIA)还是先前的化疗(pCIA),甚至是两种疗法的联合作用结果(CIA + EIA)。

三 靶向治疗、免疫治疗和干细胞移植

(一)脱发、头发质地和颜色改变

1. 脱发

虽然表皮生长因子受体(EGFR)抑制剂(如厄洛替尼、阿法替尼、西妥昔单抗、帕尼单抗)常导致轻度脱发,但据报道,接受西妥昔单抗治疗的患者中有 5% 出现瘢痕性脱发,这可能是继发性毛囊炎的结果(图 3-9)。斑秃和普秃被认为是发生在接受细胞毒性 T 淋巴细胞相关抗原-4(CTLA-4)抑制剂伊匹单抗治疗的患者中的免疫相关不良事件[18]。有报道使用纳武单抗(PD-1 抑制剂)的脱发发生率为 1%。维莫德吉[19]导致 62% 的患者脱发,停用后可见持续性脱发,其临床特征为弥漫型。

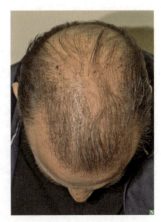

图 3-9 接受西妥昔单抗治疗患者的头皮毛囊炎

据报道在接受干细胞移植的患者中,大约 100% 的受者罹患弥漫性脱发,并伴有类似化疗所致脱发的特征。移植物抗宿主病可能导致毛发改变:急性表现包括非瘢痕性脱发,伴有弥漫性头发稀疏、斑片状脱发和头发早白。斑秃和白癜风等其他自身免疫性皮肤病已有报道。干细胞移植后的慢性移植物抗宿主病可能引起弥漫性脱发和永久性脱发,后者临床特征类似毛发扁平苔藓[20](见表 3-2)。

2. 毛发质地和色素改变

毛发质地和色素改变通常是暂时性的,直到毛囊单元调节功能重新开始正常运作(图 3-10)。毛发色素变化包括脱色(图 3-11)和再着色,最明显的是头发。据报道,多激酶抑制剂(帕唑帕尼、舒尼替尼、瑞戈非尼)可导致头发色素减退,而 EGFR 抑制剂可致头皮和面部毛发色素过度沉着(约 50%)。此外,对于接受抗 PD-1/抗 PD-L1 治疗的肺癌患者来说,头发重新着色可能是肿瘤预后良好的标志[21]。眼周区毛发过度生长、多毛症和睫毛粗长症(图 3-12)大多见于使用 EGFR 抑制剂的不良反应[22-24]。

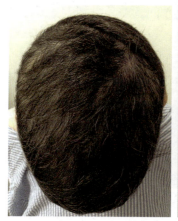
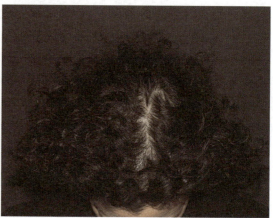

图 3-10 多柔比星和环磷酰胺化疗后患者头发质地短暂变化

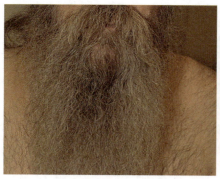
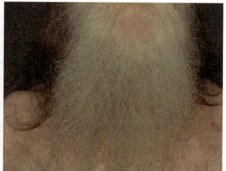

图 3-11 接受伊匹单抗/纳武单抗治疗的患者头发变白

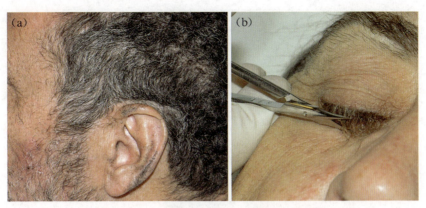

图 3-12 接受厄洛替尼治疗的患者头发变化

(a)接受厄洛替尼治疗患者的多毛症；(b)接受厄洛替尼治疗患者的睫毛粗长症。有眼部症状的患者需要修剪睫毛和眉毛，并转诊眼科。

（二）肿瘤患者毛发病症的临床分级

肿瘤学文献中已有许多方法可以客观地对毛发病症进行分级。在所有这些分级方法中，不良事件通用术语标准(CTCAE V5.0)是描述肿瘤治疗药物安全性的最常用标准（表 3-3）。其他分级方法包括世界卫生组织(WHO)、Dean 量表、美国国家癌症研究所(National Cancer Institute，NCI)和 EGFR 抑制剂皮肤毒性量表(见表 3-3)。对于睫毛和眉毛，尚无经过验证的分级标准；多毛症和睫毛粗长症用 CTCAE V5.0[25]进行分级。改良 Ferriman-Gallwey 评分(MFG 评分，多毛症评分)也可用于分级[26]。

表 3-3 抗肿瘤治疗所致毛发改变的分级评估量表

	1级	2级	3级	4级
1. 脱发分级(CTCAE V5.0)				
	脱发量＜50%正常量，远看不明显，仅在近距离观察时明显；可能需要改变发型来掩饰脱发，但不需使用假发片或假发遮盖	脱发显而易见，脱发量≥50%正常量；如果患者希望完全掩饰脱发，需要使用假发片或假发；影响社交、心理	—	—
2. 抗肿瘤治疗相关脱发 Dean 分级量表				
	＜25%脱发	25%~50%脱发	50%~75%脱发	75%~100%脱发
3. WHO 肿瘤治疗结果报告手册				
	轻度脱发	中度，局部脱发	完全脱发，但可逆	不可逆性脱发

(续表)

1级	2级	3级	4级
4. EGFR抑制剂皮肤毒性工具（MESTT）			
脱发量＜50%正常量,其他人可能会注意到,患者自觉脱发增多和总体发量减少。可能需要改变发型来掩饰脱发,但不需使用假发片或假发	2A:与健康人相比脱发量显著增多,脱发量为50%～74%正常量。脱发显而易见,很难通过改变发型来掩饰,可能要使用假发片	—	—
	2B:与正常人相比头发明显脱落,脱发量＞75%正常量,除非佩戴假发否则无法完全掩饰,或者出现新发的活检明确的瘢痕性脱发覆盖至少5%头皮面积。可能影响社交、个人生活和工作	—	—
5. 多毛症分级（CTCAE V5.0）			
毛发长度、粗细或密度增加,患者可以通过定期剃发或脱毛来掩饰,或者使用任何方式脱毛而无心理负担	至少在身体常暴露的部位（面部,不限于胡须/八字胡区域；前臂屈/伸侧）毛发长度、粗细或密度增加,需要经常剃发或破坏毛囊地脱毛来掩饰；影响社交、心理	—	—
6. 女性多毛症分级（CTCAE V5.0）			
女性患者呈现男性模式的毛发长度、粗细或密度增加,可以通过定期剃发、漂白或脱毛来掩饰	女性患者呈现男性模式的毛发长度、粗细或密度增加,需要每天剃发或持续破坏毛囊地脱毛来掩饰；影响社交、心理	—	—

四 结语

抗肿瘤治疗所致的毛发病症对肿瘤患者的生活质量产生重大影响。越来越多的证据表明,各种脱发的分子生物学基础是不同的,并且受个体易感性的影响,但它们似乎激活或共享几种分子损伤应答通路。头皮冷却似乎是预防化疗所致脱发这一特定不良事件最有希望的方法。然而，仍需要开发毛囊干细胞疗法和研究个体化风险预测策略。

参 考 文 献

1. Lemieux J, Maunsell E, Provencher L. Chemotherapy-induced alopecia and effects on quality of life among women with breast cancer: A literature review. *Psychooncology* 2008;17:317-28.
2. Kinahan KE et al. Scarring, disfigurement, and quality of life in long-term survivors of childhood cancer: A report from the Childhood Cancer Survivor study. *J Clin Oncol* 2012;30:2466-74.
3. Kang D et al. 80P — Incidence of permanent chemotherapy-induced alopecia among breast cancer patients: A five-year prospective cohort study. *Ann Oncol* 2017;28(Suppl 10).
4. Yun SJ, Kim SJ. Hair loss pattern due to chemotherapy-induced anagen effluvium: A cross-sectional observation. *Dermatology* 2007;215:36-40.
5. Paus R, Haslam IS, Sharov AA, Botchkarev VA. Pathobiology of chemotherapy-induced hair loss. *Lancet Oncol* 2013;14: e50-9.
6. Bourgeois HP et al. Long term persistent alopecia and suboptimal hair regrowth after adjuvant chemotherapy for breast cancer: Alert for an emerging side effect: French ALOPERS observatory. *Ann Oncol* 2010;21: viii83-4.
7. Sedlacek SM. Persistent significant alopecia (PSA) from adjuvant docetaxel after doxorubicin/cyclophosphamide (AC) chemotherapy in women with breast cancer. *Breast Cancer Res Treat* 2006; 171(3):627-34, abstract no. 2105.
8. Basilio FM, Brenner FM, Werner B, Rastelli GJ. Clinical and histological study of permanent alopecia after bone marrow transplantation. *Anais Brasileiros de Dermatologia* 2015;90:814-21.
9. Miteva M, Misciali C, Fanti PA, Vincenzi C, Romanelli P, Tosti A. Permanent alopecia after systemic chemotherapy: A clinicopathological study of 10 cases. *Am J Dermatopathol* 2011; 33: 345-50.
10. Tosti A, Piraccini BM, Vincenzi C, Misciali C. Permanent alopecia after busulfan chemotherapy. *Br J Dermatol* 2005;152:1056-8.
11. Haruna F, Lipsett A, Marignol L. Topical management of acute radiation dermatitis in breast cancer patients: A systematic review and meta-analysis. *Anticancer Res* 2017;37:5343-53.
12. Mubki T, Rudnicka L, Olszewska M, Shapiro J. Evaluation and diagnosis of the hair loss patient: Part I. History and clinical examination. *J Am Acad Dermatol* 2014;71:415. e1-415. e15.
13. Freites-Martinez A et al. CME Part 2: Hair disorders in cancer survivors Persistent chemotherapy-induced alopecia, persistent radiotherapy-induced alopecia, and hair growth disorders related to endocrine therapy or cancer surgery. *J Am Acad Dermatol* 2018.
14. Saggar V, Wu S, Dickler MN, Lacouture ME. Alopecia with endocrine therapies in patients with cancer. *Oncologist* 2013;18:1126-34.
15. Freites-Martinez A et al. Endocrine therapy-induced alopecia in patients with breast cancer. *JAMA Dermatology* 2018;154(6):670-5.
16. Freites-Martinez A et al. Dermatologic adverse events in breast cancer patients receiving endocrine therapies. *J Clin Oncol* 2017;35(15): e12533.
17. Al-Niaimi F, Lyon C. Tamoxifen-induced hirsutism. *J Drugs Dermatol* 2011;10:799-801.
18. Yamazaki N et al. Phase II study of ipilimumab monotherapy in Japanese patients with advanced melanoma. *Cancer Chemother Pharmacol* 2015;76:997-1004.
19. Alkeraye S, Maire C, Desmedt E, Templier C, Mortier L. Persistent alopecia induced by vismodegib.

Br J Dermatol 2015;172:1671-2.
20. Harries MJ et al. How not to get scar(r)ed: Pointers to the correct diagnosis in patients with suspected primary cicatricial alopecia. *Br J Dermatol* 2009;160:482-501.
21. Rivera N et al. Hair repigmentation during immunotherapy treatment with an anti-programmed cell death 1 and anti-programmed cell death ligand 1 agent for lung cancer. *JAMA Dermatology* 2017;153(11):1162-5.
22. Dueland S, Sauer T, Lund-Johansen F, Ostenstad B, Tveit KM. Epidermal growth factor receptor inhibition induces trichomegaly. *Acta Oncologica* 2003;42:345-6.
23. Bouche O, Brixi-Benmansour H, Bertin A, Perceau G, Lagarde S. Trichomegaly of the eyelashes following treatment with cetuximab. *Ann Oncol* 2005;16:1711-2.
24. Pascual JC, Banuls J, Belinchon I, Blanes M, Massuti B. Trichomegaly following treatment with gefitinib (ZD1839). *Br J Dermatol* 2004;151:1111-2.
25. Chen AP et al. Grading dermatologic adverse events of cancer treatments: The Common Terminology Criteria for Adverse Events Version 4.0. *J Am Acad Dermatol* 2012;67:1025-39.
26. Hatch R, Rosenfield RL, Kim MH, Tredway D. Hirsutism: Implications, etiology, and management. *Am J Obstet Gynecol* 1981;140:815-30.

第四章

光敏和光反应

赛西莉亚·拉罗卡(Cecilia A. Larocca),麦肯齐·阿塞尔(Mackenzie Asel),
马克奥·拉库蒂尔(Mario E. Lacouture)

齐思思 译

多种肿瘤治疗会引起光敏性皮疹。这种皮肤毒性被认定在不良事件通用术语标准(CTCAE)中,后者是美国国家癌症研究所(NCI)为报告肿瘤临床试验而制定的。光敏(photosensitivity)被定义为"一种以皮肤对光的敏感性增加为特征的疾病"。在许多情况下,并没有描述光敏的机制,因为这超出了临床试验的范围,也没有被CTCAE进一步定义。

光反应类型的分类通常依赖于接下来描述的主要临床和组织学特征(表4-1)[1-4]。皮肤损伤最常见的机制是光毒性反应(phototoxic reaction)。光敏性皮疹的其他亚型包括光诱导的甲分离、假性卟啉症和光过敏[1]。但是,皮疹之间可能存在明显的重叠。此外,引起光毒性皮疹的药物也可能引起光敏性皮疹。因为新的靶向药物和免疫治疗可引起光敏性皮疹,所以很可能存在其他的光敏机制,挑战当前的光生物学概念。因此,在本章中,当皮疹机制未知时,药物被统称为光敏剂。

表4-1 光反应的特征

光反应类型	紫外线暴露后发作时间	需要预先致敏	临床特征	组织学
光毒性反应	数分钟至数小时	不需要	过度的晒伤	角化不良和角质形成细胞空泡化,真皮乳头水肿,内皮细胞活化,中性粒细胞和淋巴细胞混合浸润
光敏性皮疹	数小时至数天	需要[a]	急性、亚急性、慢性炎;皮疹可能蔓延到曝光区域之外	海绵水肿,可能存在界面或苔藓样炎症模式[b]
假性卟啉症	数分钟至数小时	不需要	大疱性皮疹,继发粟丘疹、瘢痕	表皮下大疱,血管周围稀疏淋巴细胞浸润,血管壁增厚
色素沉着	数分钟至数天	不需要	呈光分布的色素沉着,伴或不伴先前的晒伤反应	噬色素细胞;真皮内Fontana染色呈阳性;某些情况下Perls染色呈阳性
光诱导的甲分离	数天(>14 d)	不需要	甲板远端裂开	不适用
光回忆性皮炎	不适用	不适用	晒伤样反应	角化不良和角质形成细胞空泡化

a:在发生光过敏之前,通常接受了数天肿瘤治疗;b:尚不清楚界面和/或苔藓样炎症是否是光过敏反应所特有的。

治疗包括严格的光保护、冷敷,并且在观察到严重程度≥2 级的特定病例中,可能需要外用和口服类固醇激素。如果通过支持性护理和严格的光保护可以充分控制症状,则光敏不是继续治疗的禁忌证。

一 光毒性反应

光毒性反应在紫外线(ultraviolet,UV)暴露后数分钟至数小时内发生[1]。并不需要事先药物暴露来致敏。这些反应可以发生在任何个体中,并且取决于药物剂量、光敏剂作用光谱中光照的强度和持续时间[5]。根据分子量,每种化学物质有其特定的作用光谱,即光被吸收后会产生激发态的波长范围。在使用维罗非尼的病例中,光毒性皮疹是由紫外线 A(UVA)暴露触发[6]。当返回到较低能量状态时,能量以热、自由基形成、荧光、磷光或电荷转移的形式释放,从而引起组织损伤[5]。炎症在晒伤反应中也起着关键作用。一种这样的介质是非编码 RNA,它在吸收能量后与 Toll 样受体结合以触发炎症反应[7]。此外,某些抗癌剂(例如紫杉烷)通过间接产生卟啉引起光毒性皮疹[1,8,9]。这些病例的临床表现(图 4-1、图 4-2)与经典的光毒性反应无法区分;没有见到卟啉症的临床和组织学特征。另外,靶向治疗可能通过干扰对紫外线介导损伤的正常细胞反应,引起过度晒伤样反应(表 4-2)。

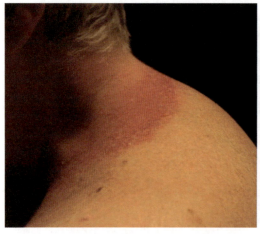

图 4-1 维罗非尼的 UVA 诱导性光毒性皮疹

患者出现界限清晰的弥漫性红斑,仅影响曝光部位,衣服覆盖区域未受累。

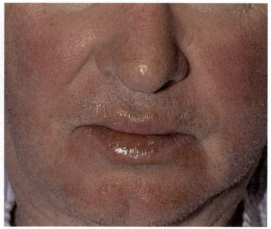

图 4-2 维罗非尼引起的光毒性皮疹,曝光部位出现红斑和水疱

(经 John Wiley & Sons Inc. 许可发表,Lacouture M E, et al. Oncologist,2013,18:3.)

表 4-2 光毒性反应的诱导剂

化疗药物	靶向药
达卡巴嗪	达拉非尼
放线菌素	伊马替尼
多柔比星	来那度胺
氟尿嘧啶	凡德他尼
羟基脲	维罗非尼
丝裂霉素 C	维 A 酸类药物（阿维 A 酯、异维 A 酸）
丙卡巴肼	
替加氟	
硫鸟嘌呤	
长春碱	
卡培他滨＋白蛋白结合型紫杉醇	

注：更多信息见参考文献 6、8、11-27。

临床表现和组织学表现是晒伤反应，在曝光部位出现融合性红斑[1]。在严重情况下，水疱和大疱可能在紫外线暴露后 24~48 h 出现。随着时间的推移，皮肤会出现晒黑伴片状脱屑。最常见的曝光部位是面部和颈部，不包括鼻唇沟、上眼睑皱褶、面部和颈部的深沟以及受头发、耳朵和鼻子阴影保护的区域。在身体上，衣服覆盖区和曝光部位皮肤之间有明显的分界，红斑通常局限在胸部"V"形区、前臂伸侧和手背[1]。

使用舒缓的外用润肤剂进行支持性治疗。然而，炎症广泛（水肿、红斑、疼痛）的情况下，可以考虑外用和/或口服类固醇激素。虽然光敏不是继续治疗的禁忌证，但对于某些药物如达卡巴嗪而言，光毒性反应的严重度可能随着持续暴露而恶化。对于无法遵循严格光保护的患者，需要减少剂量和停止治疗[10]。

有几种光毒性皮疹的变异（表 4-3、表 4-4）[1]。光回忆性皮炎是指给药后引起光毒性皮疹再次出现。使用甲氨蝶呤时，如果在紫外线暴露后数天开始用药，则会引起光回忆性皮炎。因此，在前 1 周内发生过晒伤、接受过光疗或放疗的患者可能需要推迟使用甲氨蝶呤[28]。目前尚不清楚紫杉烷是否会诱发真正的紫外线回忆性皮炎，因为它与另一种更常见的紫杉烷相关毒性相似，后者称之为关节周围红斑伴甲分离（PATEO），它与光反应一样，出现在手背上。一些病例在曝光部位出现色素沉着[1,11]。色素沉着可能在日晒后立即出现，或者在治疗数天后作为延迟反应出现，而在这之前没有明显的红斑性晒伤皮疹。光诱导的甲分离被认为是由于光敏影响到甲床，在紫外线暴露后 2 周或更长时间内出现[1,11]。

表 4-3 光毒性变异反应的诱导剂

光毒性反应	化疗药	靶向药
光诱导的甲分离[8,11,29,30]	巯嘌呤 紫杉醇	凡德他尼 维罗非尼
光回忆性皮炎[11,31-35]	吉西他滨 多西紫杉醇 甲氨蝶呤 紫杉醇 培美曲塞 苏拉明 多西他赛-环磷酰胺 依托泊苷-环磷酰胺 甲氨蝶呤-环磷酰胺-氟尿嘧啶	索拉非尼
色素沉着(呈光分布)[11,36,37]	柔红霉素 多柔比星 氟尿嘧啶 羟基脲 普卡霉素	凡德他尼 维罗非尼

表 4-4 光敏性皮疹的诱导剂[a]

抗癌药	临床特征	发作时间[b]	组织学
化疗药			
表柔比星-博来霉素-长春新碱[38]	暴露在阳光下的腿部在数小时内出现瘙痒,抓挠部位出现水肿性红色斑块,48 h后进展为大疱;仅表柔比星的光斑贴试验阳性	第一次持续输注表柔比星、博来霉素和长春新碱治疗的当天	棘层肥厚,海绵水肿,淋巴、组织细胞浸润伴嗜酸性粒细胞
卡培他滨[39-41]	躯干和四肢曝光部位呈紫色至红色平顶丘疹或斑块,伴有脱屑;1例有甲周红斑及脱屑	2周至2个月	界面皮炎伴苔藓样或基底细胞空泡化改变,偶见角质形成细胞坏死,血管周围淋巴细胞浸润
替加氟[42,43]	光暴露部位日晒后24 h,出现红色扁平苔藓样皮疹;其他报道湿疹样皮炎	2年	界面皮炎,血管周围单核细胞浸润
白蛋白结合型紫杉醇[44,45]	面部、胸部、前臂曝光部位出现融合性红斑,伴有脱屑和色素沉着,境界清晰	1个月	角化过度、轻度棘层肥厚、海绵水肿、稀疏的界面皮炎和色素失禁
羟基脲[46]	曝光部位瘙痒性红斑、丘疹和斑块	不适用	非干酪坏死的结节病样肉芽肿

(续表)

抗癌药	临床特征	发作时间	组织学
靶向药			
特司林-洛伐妥珠单抗[47]	光敏感,在临床试验中没有更多的特征;晒后数小时出现晒伤样反应(个例)	1周	不适用
伊马替尼[48]	晒伤样;3个月后出现口腔黏膜蕾丝状白色条纹	1年	皮肤和黏膜的界面皮炎
索拉非尼[49]	光敏感,在临床试验中没有更多的特征		
凡德他尼[37,50-54]	呈光分布的瘙痒性苔藓样皮炎;3例出现疼痛或瘙痒的晒伤样反应,伴有水疱、糜烂,后形成苔藓样鳞屑性斑块	1~24周	不同程度的苔藓样淋巴细胞浸润,海绵水肿,角质形成细胞凋亡
	呈光分布的靶样病变:多形红斑;光斑贴试验阳性	3周	空泡化界面皮炎、轻度海绵水肿、角质形成细胞变性、血管周围和间质内淋巴细胞和嗜酸性粒细胞浸润
	曝光后2周,在光暴露部位出现几乎融合的瘙痒性湿疹样红色斑块伴水疱	1个月	浅丛血管周围性皮炎,伴嗜酸性粒细胞浸润和局灶海绵水肿
氟他胺[11,55]	曝光部位出现丘疹水疱红斑或脱屑;1例进展为红皮病;部分光斑贴试验阳性	2~5个月	不适用
免疫治疗			
纳武单抗[56] 帕博利珠单抗[57] 伊匹单抗[58]	光敏感,未提供进一步描述	不适用	不适用

a:表中包括的病例,有未描述光敏性机制的,有光过敏的,或者具有光过敏和光毒性的重叠特征;b:皮疹发作前肿瘤治疗的持续时间。

二 光过敏反应

光过敏反应(photoallergic reaction)需要事先暴露致敏,因此通常在抗癌治疗数天后出现皮疹,一般在14 d内[1,28]。临床上,这些皮疹表现为湿疹样皮炎(图4-3、图4-4);组织学上可见海绵水肿[1,5,28]。这是肿瘤治疗中少见的皮肤毒性。

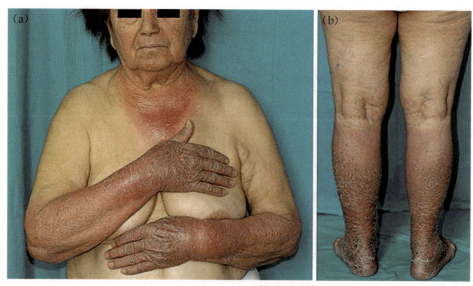

图4-3 凡德他尼引起的光过敏反应

位于头颈部、肩部、双侧前臂(a)和腿部(b)的红色水肿性鳞屑性皮损
经 John Wiley & Sons Inc. 许可再发表。Fava P, et al. Dermatol Ther, 2010, 23:5。

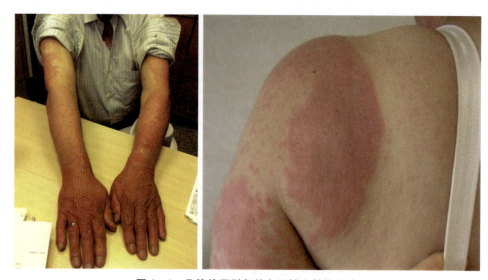

图4-4 凡德他尼引起的多形性光敏性皮疹

经 Grande E 等许可引用。凡德他尼治疗晚期甲状腺髓样癌：不良事件管理策略的综述。
Springer Nature；Springer Nature, Advances in Therapy, 2013。

具有多形红斑、界面皮炎、苔藓样或肉芽肿性皮炎组织学表现的呈光分布的皮疹是否代表一种真正的光过敏，还是肿瘤治疗对皮肤直接或间接影响的反映，现在尚不清楚。

三、光照加重的疾病

肿瘤治疗可能导致皮肤病因暴露于紫外线辐射而加重（表4-5）。据报道，化疗、靶向治疗和免疫治疗均可诱发结缔组织病，例如亚急性皮肤型红斑狼疮这一光敏性自身免疫性疾病[59-63]。特别是羟基脲，它与多种光敏性结缔组织疾病有关，是药物性皮肌炎最常见的诱因[64-66]。替加氟还引起皮肌炎和狼疮样综合征[11]。

表4-5 光照性皮肤病的诱导剂

疾病	化疗	靶向治疗	其他治疗
亚急性皮肤红斑狼疮	卡培他滨[59,61,70,71] 多西他赛[60] 多柔比星[72] 氟尿嘧啶[73] 吉西他滨[62] 羟基脲[64] 米托坦[74] 紫杉醇[75] 多柔比星-环磷酰胺[72] 氟尿嘧啶-卡培他滨[76]		亮丙瑞林[77] 纳武单抗[63] 他莫昔芬[78] 凡德替尼[37]
痤疮样皮疹		EGFR 抑制剂[10]	
卟啉症	白消安[11] 苯丁酸氮芥[79] 顺铂[80] 环磷酰胺[81] 氟尿嘧啶[82] 甲氨蝶呤[83]	氟他胺[84-86] 伊马替尼[87,88]	
药物诱导的糙皮病	巯嘌呤[1] 氟尿嘧啶[1]		

表皮生长因子受体（EGFR）抑制剂会在大多数患者中引起皮肤毒性。众所周知，其与丘疹脓疱性皮疹相关（图4-5）。有趣的是，一些患者的丘疹脓疱性皮疹会被紫外线诱发或加重[67]。EGFR 抑制剂引起的皮疹通常发生于曝光部位，包括面部、上背部和胸部"V"形区。皮疹的严重程度与 Fitzpatrick 皮肤类型相关。Ⅰ～Ⅱ型皮肤患者3级或更高级别皮疹的发生率为63%，而Ⅲ～Ⅳ型皮肤为5%，Ⅴ～Ⅵ型皮肤为0%[10]。这种相关性可能与EGFR 信号在角质形成细胞抵御紫外线辐射诱导的凋亡和氧化应激中的保护作用有关，这一点已在体外得到证实[68,69]。

多种化疗药物会诱发卟啉症[3,11]。药物性卟啉症是一种呈光分布的大疱性疾病，在没有卟啉异常的情况下具有迟发性皮肤卟啉症的临床和组织学特征（水疱、大疱、皮肤脆性增

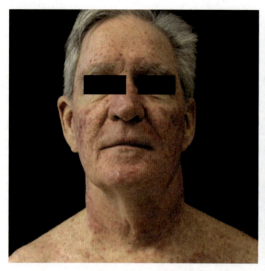 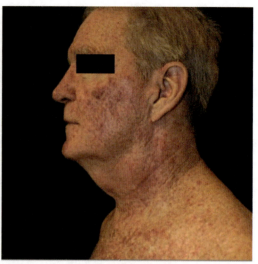

图 4-5　EGFR 抑制剂引起的痤疮样皮疹发作，见于面颈部曝光区域

注意下颌下方的皮肤不受累，下颈部患者衬衫衣领处境界清晰的红斑。

加、粟丘疹和瘢痕）[3]。

糙皮病是一种由烟酸缺乏引起的光敏性皮炎，表现为红斑性晒伤，随后出现皮肤增厚、色素沉着和羊皮纸样脱屑[5]。与正常的晒伤相比，其从光损伤中恢复需要更长的时间。选择性化疗通过干扰烟酸的生物合成而引起糙皮病[1]。

四　光分布性疾病

抗癌治疗引起的皮肤毒性反应呈光分布时可能与光敏性皮疹相混淆，但它们反映的是既往的光损伤史。一个常见的例子是日光性角化病的炎症反应（图 4-6，表 4-6）。通常在化疗开始后 1 周内，在既往已有日光性角化病的部位出现红斑、瘙痒和角化过度增加[11]。此外，已报道多种肿瘤治疗后出现苔藓样皮疹。目前尚不清楚它们究竟是光照后加重，还是仅仅为光分布。在 PD-1 抑制剂引起的苔藓样皮炎病例中，窄谱 UVB 已被用于治疗，这反驳了潜在的光敏性[89]。

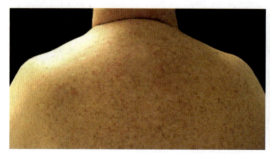 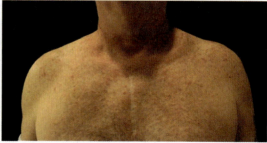

图 4-6　呈光分布的炎症性日光性角化病

患者的炎症性日光性角化病主要位于上胸部和背部的曝光区域。

表4-6 日光性角化病的炎症反应

化 疗 药	其他治疗
卡培他滨	厄洛替尼
卡铂	索拉非尼
顺铂	索拉非尼-替比法尼
达卡巴嗪	纳武单抗
放线菌素	帕博利珠单抗
脱氧可福霉素	
多西他赛	
多柔比星	
氟达拉滨	
氟尿嘧啶	
紫杉醇	
喷司他丁	
长春新碱	
放线菌素-达卡巴嗪-长春新碱	
多柔比星-阿糖胞苷-硫鸟嘌呤	
多柔比星-长春新碱	

注：更多信息见参考文献 11、90—95。

五 结语

化疗、靶向治疗和免疫治疗，无论作用机制如何，均可诱发光敏性皮疹。抗癌治疗中最常引起光敏的原因是维罗非尼，＞50%的患者出现皮疹[6,17,96,97]。除维罗非尼外，凡德他尼也常与光敏性皮疹相关，＞37%的患者出现皮疹[37,98,99]。有趣的是，凡德他尼已被证实可诱导多种不同的光敏性皮疹，与光毒性和光过敏现象一致。临床表现不一，包括过度晒伤、呈光分布的苔藓样皮疹、抗核抗体升高的亚急性皮肤狼疮、光诱导的多形红斑伴光斑贴试验阳性、呈光分布的蓝灰色色素沉着和光诱导的甲分离[13,15,30,36,37,50-53]。与凡德他尼一样，氟尿嘧啶也能够诱导多种光反应[1,3,11,73]。

在开始肿瘤治疗之前，进行有关光保护的前期教育对于减轻这些反应至关重要。此外，鉴于某些药物的半衰期长，即使在停用致病药物后继续光保护也是明智之举。对于1级事件，外用类固醇激素和抗组胺药的支持性治疗是令人满意的。≥2级事件可能需要系统使用类固醇激素。同样重要的是认识到，患者也可能在使用其他光敏性药物，如抗生素、利尿剂或非甾体抗炎药（NSAID）[28]。

参 考 文 献

1. Gould JW, Mercurio MG, Elmets CA. Cutaneous photosensitivity diseases induced by exogenous agents. *J Am Acad Dermatol* 1995;33(4):551-73, quiz 74-76.
2. Gilchrest BA, Soter NA, Stoff JS, Mihm MC Jr. The human sunburn reaction: Histologic and biochemical studies. *J Am Acad Dermatol* 1981;5(4):411-22.

3. Green JJ, Manders SM. Pseudoporphyria. *J Am Acad Dermatol* 2001;44(1):100-8.
4. Rhodes LE et al. The sunburn response in human skin is characterized by sequential eicosanoid profiles that may mediate its early and late phases. *FASEB J* 2009;23(11):3947-56.
5. James WD, Elston DM, Berger TG, Andrews GC, editors. *Andrews' Diseases of the Skin: Clinical Dermatology*. London: Saunders/Elsevier; 2011.
6. Dummer R, Rinderknecht J, Goldinger SM. Ultraviolet A and photosensitivity during vemurafenib therapy. *N Engl J Med* 2012;366(5):480-1.
7. Bernard JJ et al. Ultraviolet radiation damages self noncoding RNA and is detected by TLR3. *Nat Med* 2012;18(8):1286-90.
8. Cohen AD et al. Cutaneous photosensitivity induced by paclitaxel and trastuzumab therapy associated with aberrations in the biosynthesis of porphyrins. *J Dermatolog Treat* 2005;16(1):19-21.
9. Akay BN, Unlu E, Buyukcelik A, Akyol A. Photosensitive rash in association with porphyrin biosynthesis possibly induced by docetaxel and trastuzumab therapy in a patient with metastatic breast carcinoma. *Jpn J Clin Oncol* 2010;40(10):989-91.
10. Lacouture ME, editor. *Dermatologic Principles and Practice in Oncology: Conditions of the Skin, Hair and Nails in Cancer Patients*. 1st ed. Hoboken, NJ: John Wiley & Sons; 2007.
11. Susser WS, Whitaker-Worth DL, Grant-Kels JM. Mucocutaneous reactions to chemotherapy. *J Am Acad Dermatol* 1999;40(3):367-98, quiz 399-400.
12. Scheithauer W et al. Phase II trial of capecitabine plus nab-paclitaxel in patients with metastatic pancreatic adenocarcinoma. *J Gastrointest Oncol* 2016;7(2):234-8.
13. Rosen AC, Wu S, Damse A, Sherman E, Lacouture ME. Risk of rash in cancer patients treated with vandetanib: Systematic review and meta-analysis. *J Clin Endocrinol Metab* 2012;97(4):1125-33.
14. Salvador A, Vedaldi D, Brun P, Dall'Acqua S. Vandetanib-induced phototoxicity in human keratinocytes NCTC-2544. *Toxicol In Vitro* 2014;28(5):803-11.
15. Son YM, Roh JY, Cho EK, Lee JR. Photosensitivity reactions to vandetanib: Redevelopment after sequential treatment with docetaxel. *Ann Dermatol* 2011;23(Suppl 3): S314-8.
16. Boudewijns S, Gerritsen WR, Koornstra RH. Case series: Indoor-photosensitivity caused by fluorescent lamps in patients treated with vemurafenib for metastatic melanoma. *BMC Cancer* 2014;14:967.
17. Boussemart L et al. Prospective study of cutaneous side-effects associated with the BRAF inhibitor vemurafenib: A study of 42 patients. *Ann Oncol* 2013;24(6):1691-7.
18. Brugiere C et al. Vemurafenib skin phototoxicity is indirectly linked to ultraviolet A minimal erythema dose decrease. *Br J Dermatol* 2014;171(6):1529-32.
19. Gabeff R et al. Phototoxicity of B-RAF inhibitors: Exclusively due to UVA radiation and rapidly regressive. *Eur J Dermatol* 2015;25(5):452-6.
20. Woods JA et al. The phototoxicity of vemurafenib: An investigation of clinical monochromator phototesting and *in vitro* phototoxicity testing. *J Photochem Photobiol B* 2015;151:233-8.
21. Carlos G et al. Cutaneous toxic effects of BRAF inhibitors alone and in combination with MEK inhibitors for metastatic melanoma. *JAMA Dermatol* 2015;151(10):1103-9.
22. Brouard M, Saurat JH. Cutaneous reactions to STI571. *N Engl J Med* 2001;345(8):618-9.
23. Liu W et al. The tyrosine kinase inhibitor imatinib mesylate enhances the efficacy of photodynamic therapy by inhibiting ABCG2. *Clin Cancer Res* 2007;13(8):2463-70.
24. Nardi G, Lhiaubet-Vallet V, Miranda MA. Photosensitization by imatinib. A photochemical and photobiological study of the drug and its substructures. *Chem Res Toxicol* 2014;27(11):1990-5.
25. Valeyrie L et al. Adverse cutaneous reactions to imatinib (STI571) in Philadelphia chromosome-

positive leukemias: A prospective study of 54 patients. *J Am Acad Dermatol* 2003;48(2):201-6.
26. Perez-Paredes MG, Rodriguez-Prieto MA, Ruiz-Gonzalez I, Valladares-Narganes LM. Lenalidomide-induced photosensitivity. *Photodermatol Photoimmunol Photomed* 2013;29(6):334-6.
27. Ferguson J, Johnson BE. Retinoid associated phototoxicity and photosensitivity. *Pharmacol Ther* 1989;40(1):123-35.
28. Monteiro AF, Rato M, Martins C. Drug-induced photosensitivity: Photoallergic and phototoxic reactions. *Clin Dermatol* 2016;34(5):571-81.
29. Hussain S, Anderson DN, Salvatti ME, Adamson B, McManus M, Braverman AS. Onycholysis as a complication of systemic chemotherapy: Report of five cases associated with prolonged weekly paclitaxel therapy and review of the literature. *Cancer* 2000;88(10):2367-71.
30. Negulescu M et al. Development of photoonycholysis with vandetanib therapy. *Skin Appendage Disord* 2017;2(3-4):146-51.
31. Badger J, Kang S, Uzieblo A, Srinivas S. Double diagnosis in cancer patients and cutaneous reaction related to gemcitabine: CASE 3. Photo therapy recall with gemcitabine following ultraviolet B treatment. *J Clin Oncol* 2005;23(28):7224-5.
32. Droitcourt C, Le Ho H, Adamski H, Le Gall F, Dupuy A. Docetaxel-induced photo-recall phenomenon. *Photodermatol Photoimmunol Photomed* 2012;28(4):222-3.
33. Ee HL, Yosipovitch G. Photo recall phenomenon: An adverse reaction to taxanes. *Dermatology* 2003;207(2):196-8.
34. Basile FG, Creamer S. Docetaxel/cyclophosphamide-induced ultraviolet recall dermatitis. *Am J Clin Oncol* 2011;29(34):e840-1.
35. Magne N, Chargari C, Auberdiac P, Moncharmont C, Merrouche Y, Spano JP. Ultraviolet recall dermatitis reaction with sorafenib. *Invest New Drugs* 2011;29(5):1111-3.
36. Kong HH, Fine HA, Stern JB, Turner ML. Cutaneous pigmentation after photosensitivity induced by vandetanib therapy. *Arch Dermatol* 2009;145(8):923-5.
37. Giacchero D et al. A new spectrum of skin toxic effects associated with the multikinase inhibitor vandetanib. *Arch Dermatol* 2012;148(12):1418-20.
38. Balabanova MB. Photoprovoked erythematobullous eruption from farmorubicin. *Contact Dermatitis* 1994;30(5):303-4.
39. Hague JS, Ilchyshyn A. Lichenoid photosensitive eruption due to capecitabine chemotherapy for metastatic breast cancer. *Clin Exp Dermatol* 2007;32(1):102-3.
40. Walker G, Lane N, Parekh P. Photosensitive lichenoid drug eruption to capecitabine. *J Am Acad Dermatol* 2014;71(2):e52-3.
41. Willey A, Glusac EJ, Bolognia JL. Photoeruption in a patient treated with capecitabine (Xeloda) for metastatic breast cancer. *J Am Acad Dermatol* 2002;47(3):453.
42. Horio T, Yokoyama M. Tegaful photosensitivity — Lichenoid and eczematous types. *Photodermatol* 1986;3(3):192-3.
43. Usuki A, Funasaka Y, Oka M, Ichihashi M. Tegafur-induced photosensitivity — Evaluation of provocation by UVB irradiation. *Int J Dermatol* 1997;36(8):604-6.
44. Beutler BD, Cohen PR. Nab-paclitaxel-associated photosensitivity: Report in a woman with non-small cell lung cancer and review of taxane-related photodermatoses. *Dermatol Pract Concept* 2015;5(2):121-4.
45. Cohen PR. Photodistributed erythema multiforme: Paclitaxel-related, photosensitive conditions in patients with cancer. *J Drugs Dermatol* 2009;8(1):61-4.
46. Leon-Mateos A et al. Photo-induced granulomatous eruption by hydroxyurea. *J Eur Acad Dermatol*

Venereol 2007;21(10):1428-9.
47. Rudin CM et al. Rovalpituzumab tesirine, a DLL3-targeted antibody-drug conjugate, in recurrent small-cell lung cancer: A first-in-human, first-in-class, open-label, phase 1 study. *Lancet Oncol* 2017;18(1):42-51.
48. Brazzelli V et al. Photoinduced dermatitis and oral lichenoid reaction in a chronic myeloid leukemia patient treated with imatinib mesylate. *Photodermatol Photoimmunol Photomed* 2012;28(1):2-5.
49. Lam ET et al. Phase II clinical trial of sorafenib in metastatic medullary thyroid cancer. *Am J Clin Oncol* 2010;28(14):2323-30.
50. Caro-Gutierrez D, Floristan Muruzabal MU, Gomez de la Fuente E, Franco AP, Lopez Estebaranz JL. Photo-induced erythema multiforme associated with vandetanib administration. *J Am Acad Dermatol* 2014;71(4):e142-4.
51. Goldstein J, Patel AB, Curry JL, Subbiah V, Piha-Paul S. Photoallergic reaction in a patient receiving vandetanib for metastatic follicular thyroid carcinoma: A case report. *BMC Dermatol* 2015;15:2.
52. Bota J, Harvey V, Ferguson C, Hood A. A rare case of late-onset lichenoid photodermatitis after vandetanib therapy. *JAAD Case Rep* 2015;1(3):141-3.
53. Chang CH, Chang JW, Hui CY, Yang CH. Severe photosensitivity reaction to vandetanib. *Am J Clin Oncol* 2009;27(27):e114-5.
54. Fava P, Quaglino P, Fierro MT, Novelli M, Bernengo MG. Therapeutic hotline. A rare vandetanib-induced photo-allergic drug eruption. *Dermatol Ther* 2010;23(5):553-5.
55. Yokote R, Tokura Y, Igarashi N, Ishikawa O, Miyachi Y. Photosensitive drug eruption induced by flutamide. *Eur J Dermatol* 1998;8(6):427-9.
56. Robert C et al. Nivolumab in previously untreated melanoma without BRAF mutation. *N Engl J Med* 2015;372(4):320-30.
57. Sanlorenzo M et al. Pembrolizumab cutaneous adverse events and their association with disease progression. *JAMA Dermatol* 2015;151(11):1206-12.
58. Voskens CJ et al. The price of tumor control: An analysis of rare side effects of anti-CTLA-4 therapy in metastatic melanoma from the ipilimumab network. *PLoS One* 2013;8(1):e53745.
59. Ko JH, Hsieh CI, Chou CY, Wang KH. Capecitabine-induced subacute cutaneous lupus erythematosus: Report of a case with positive rechallenge test. *J Dermatol* 2013;40(11):939-40.
60. Chen M, Crowson AN, Woofter M, Luca MB, Magro CM. Docetaxel (taxotere) induced subacute cutaneous lupus erythematosus: Report of 4 cases. *J Rheumatol* 2004;31(4):818-20.
61. Fernandes NF, Rosenbach M, Elenitsas R, Kist JM. Subacute cutaneous lupus erythematosus associated with capecitabine monotherapy. *Arch Dermatol* 2009;145(3):340-1.
62. Wiznia LE, Subtil A, Choi JN. Subacute cutaneous lupus erythematosus induced by chemotherapy: Gemcitabine as a causative agent. *JAMA Dermatol* 2013;149(9):1071-5.
63. Liu RC, Sebaratnam DF, Jackett L, Kao S, Lowe PM. Subacute cutaneous lupus erythematosus induced by nivolumab. *Australas J Dermatol* 2017;59(2):e152-4.
64. Yanes DA, Mosser-Goldfarb JL. A cutaneous lupus erythematosus-like eruption induced by hydroxyurea. *Pediatr Dermatol* 2017;34(1):e30-1.
65. Seidler AM, Gottlieb AB. Dermatomyositis induced by drug therapy: A review of case reports. *J Am Acad Dermatol* 2008;59(5):872-80.
66. Layton AM, Cotterill JA, Tomlinson IW. Hydroxyurea-induced lupus erythematosus. *Br J Dermatol* 1994;130(5):687-8.
67. Luu M, Lai SE, Patel J, Guitart J, Lacouture ME. Photosensitive rash due to the epidermal growth factor receptor inhibitor erlotinib. *Photodermatol Photoimmunol Photomed* 2007;23(1):42-5.

68. Peus D, Vasa RA, Meves A, Beyerle A, Pittelkow MR. UVB-induced epidermal growth factor receptor phosphorylation is critical for downstream signaling and keratinocyte survival. *Photochem Photobiol* 2000;72(1):135-40.
69. El-Abaseri TB, Putta S, Hansen LA. Ultraviolet irradiation induces keratinocyte proliferation and epidermal hyperplasia through the activation of the epidermal growth factor receptor. *Carcinogenesis* 2006;27(2):225-31.
70. Floristan U et al. Subacute cutaneous lupus erythematosus induced by capecitabine. *Clin Exp Dermatol* 2009;34(7):e328-9.
71. Kim WI et al. Subacute cutaneous lupus erythematosus induced by capecitabine: 5-FU was innocent. *J Eur Acad Dermatol Venereol* 2016;30(11):e163-4.
72. Funke AA, Kulp-Shorten CL, Callen JP. Subacute cutaneous lupus erythematosus exacerbated or induced by chemotherapy. *Arch Dermatol* 2010;146(10):1113-6.
73. Almagro BM et al. Occurrence of subacute cutaneous lupus erythematosus after treatment with systemic fluorouracil. *Am J Clin Oncol* 2011;29(20):e613-5.
74. Mayor-Ibarguren A, Roldan-Puchalt MC, Gomez-Fernandez C, Albizuri-Prado F, Alvarez-Escola C. Subacute cutaneous lupus erythematosus induced by mitotane. *JAMA Dermatol* 2016;152(1):109-11.
75. Adachi A, Horikawa T. Paclitaxel-induced cutaneous lupus erythematosus in patients with serum anti-SSA/Ro antibody. *J Dermatol* 2007;34(7):473-6.
76. Weger W, Kranke B, Gerger A, Salmhofer W, Aberer E. Occurrence of subacute cutaneous lupus erythematosus after treatment with fluorouracil and capecitabine. *J Am Acad Dermatol* 2008;59(2 Suppl 1):S4-6.
77. Wiechert A, Tuting T, Bieber T, Haidl G, Wenzel J. Subacute cutaneous lupus erythematosus in a leuprorelin-treated patient with prostate carcinoma. *Br J Dermatol* 2008;159(1):231-3.
78. Fumal I, Danchin A, Cosserat F, Barbaud A, Schmutz JL. Subacute cutaneous lupus erythematosus associated with tamoxifen therapy: Two cases. *Dermatology* 2005;210(3):251-2.
79. Davies JH, Whitaker SJ. Chlorambucil and acute intermittent porphyria. *Clin Oncol (R Coll Radiol)* 2002;14(6):491-3.
80. Aramburo Gonzalez P, Roman Garcia FJ, Gonzalez Quintela A, Barbadillo Garcia de Velasco R. [A case of porphyria after treatment with cisplatin]. *Med Clin* 1986;87(17):738-9.
81. Manzione NC, Wolkoff AW, Sassa S. Development of porphyria cutanea tarda after treatment with cyclophosphamide. *Gastroenterology* 1988;95(4):1119-22.
82. Laidman PJ, Gebauer K, Trotter J. 5-Fluorouracil-induced pseudoporphyria. *Aust N Z J Med* 1992;22(4):385.
83. O'Neill T, Simpson J, Smyth SJ, Lovell C, Calin A. Porphyria cutanea tarda associated with methotrexate therapy. *Br J Rheumatol* 1993;32(5):411-2.
84. Schmutz JL, Barbaud A, Trechot P. [Flutamide and pseudoporphyria]. *Ann Dermatol Venereol* 1999;126(4):374.
85. Mantoux F, Bahadoran P, Perrin C, Bermon C, Lacour JP, Ortonne JP. [Flutamide-induced late cutaneous pseudoporphyria]. *Ann Dermatol Venereol* 1999;126(2):150-2.
86. Borroni G et al. Flutamide-induced pseudoporphyria. *Br J Dermatol* 1998;138(4):711-2.
87. Berghoff AT, English JC 3rd. Imatinib mesylate-induced pseudoporphyria. *J Am Acad Dermatol* 2010;63(1):e14-6.
88. Batrani M, Salhotra M, Kubba A, Agrawal M. Imatinib mesylate-induced pseudoporphyria in a patient with chronic myeloid leukemia. *Indian J Dermatol Venereol Leprol* 2016;82(6):727-9.
89. Shi VJ et al. Clinical and histologic features of lichenoid mucocutaneous eruptions due to anti-

programmed cell death 1 and anti-programmed cell death ligand 1 immunotherapy. *JAMA Dermatol* 2016;152(10):1128-36.

90. Johnson TM, Rapini RP, Duvic M. Inflammation of actinic keratoses from systemic chemotherapy. *J Am Acad Dermatol* 1987;17(2 Pt 1):192-7.

91. Hermanns JF, Pierard GE, Quatresooz P. Erlotinib-responsive actinic keratoses. *Oncol Rep* 2007;18(3):581-4.

92. Lewis KG, Lewis MD, Robinson-Bostom L, Pan TD. Inflammation of actinic keratoses during capecitabine therapy. *Arch Dermatol* 2004;140(3):367-8.

93. Ali FR, Yiu ZZ, Fitzgerald D. Inflammation of actinic keratoses during paclitaxel chemotherapy. *BMJ Case Rep* 2015;2015.

94. Hardwick N, Murray A. Inflammation of actinic keratoses induced by cytotoxic drugs. *Br J Dermatol* 1986;114(5):639-40.

95. Lacouture ME et al. Inflammation of actinic keratoses subsequent to therapy with sorafenib, a multitargeted tyrosine-kinase inhibitor. *Clin Exp Dermatol* 2006;31(6):783-5.

96. Sanlorenzo M et al. Comparative profile of cutaneous adverse events: BRAF/MEK inhibitor combination therapy versus BRAF monotherapy in melanoma. *J Am Acad Dermatol* 2014;71(6):1102-9. e1.

97. Sosman JA et al. Survival in BRAF V600-mutant advanced melanoma treated with vemurafenib. *N Engl J Med* 2012;366(8):707-14.

98. Kharfan-Dabaja MA et al. Clinical practice recommendations on indication and timing of hematopoietic cell transplantation in mature T cell and NK/T cell lymphomas: An international collaborative effort on behalf of the guidelines committee of the American Society for Blood and Marrow Transplantation. *Biol Blood Marrow Transplant* 2017;23(11):1826-38.

99. Leboulleux S et al. Vandetanib in locally advanced or metastatic differentiated thyroid cancer: A randomised, double-blind, phase 2 trial. *Lancet Oncol* 2012;13(9):897-905.

第五章

角化过度性反应

文森特·西博(Vincent Sibaud),玛丽亚·瓦斯塔雷拉(Maria Vastarella)

胡瑞铭 译

继发的角化过度性反应常报道与系统性抗肿瘤治疗有关。这通常见于酪氨酸激酶抑制剂,也可见于细胞毒性化疗药物和新获批的免疫检查点抑制剂(ICI)。药物破坏表皮稳态、与角质形成细胞增殖/分化或生存相互作用,可导致各种角化过度性反应,包括手足皮肤反应、诱导性银屑病、毛周角化病或毛发红糠疹样皮疹、暂时性棘层松解性皮肤病(Grover病)、接触性角化过度症和鳞状上皮增生性皮肤肿瘤(表5-1)。

表5-1 抗肿瘤治疗相关的主要角化过度性反应

角化过度性反应	主 要 致 病 药 物
手足皮肤反应	多激酶血管生成抑制剂(索拉非尼、瑞戈非尼、阿西替尼、舒尼替尼、卡博替尼±帕唑帕尼) 选择性BRAF抑制剂[a](维罗非尼、达拉非尼、康奈非尼)
银屑病	化疗药物 血管生成抑制剂(贝伐珠单抗、舒尼替尼、索拉非尼) 抗CD20单抗(利妥昔单抗) Bcr-Abi抑制剂(伊马替尼、尼洛替尼) α-干扰素 免疫检查点抑制剂(抗PD-1、抗CTLA-4)
疣状角化病	选择性BRAF抑制剂[a]
鳞状细胞癌和角化棘皮瘤	选择性BRAF抑制剂[a] 泛RAF抑制剂(索拉非尼、瑞戈非尼) 免疫检查点抑制剂(抗PD-1) 化疗药物(羟基脲、氟达拉滨)
炎症性日光性角化病/脂溢性角化病	化疗药物(5-氟尿嘧啶、卡培他滨、紫杉醇类、顺铂等) 选择性BRAF抑制剂[a] 免疫检查点抑制剂
毛发角化病样皮疹	Bcr-Abi抑制剂(达沙替尼、尼洛替尼、普纳替尼) 选择性BRAF抑制剂和泛RAF抑制剂

(续表)

角化过度性反应	主要致病药物
毛发红糠疹样皮疹	普纳替尼 索拉非尼
暂时性棘层松解性皮肤病（Grover 病）	选择性 BRAF 抑制剂[a] 免疫检查点抑制剂 化疗、放疗、内分泌治疗药物
其他损害（囊性病变、接触性角化过度症、寻常疣）	选择性 BRAF 抑制剂[a] ± 泛 RAF 抑制剂

a：单药治疗。与 MEK 抑制剂联合使用，可显著抑制发生角化过度性病变。

一 手足皮肤反应

（一）多激酶血管生成抑制剂

手足皮肤反应（HFSR）是最常见的、剂量限制的、临床上显著的皮肤不良事件，常见于接受多激酶血管生成抑制剂（如索拉非尼、瑞戈非尼、阿西替尼、卡博替尼、舒尼替尼、帕唑帕尼）治疗的患者，该抑制剂同时靶向血管内皮生长因子受体（VEGFR）和血小板衍生生长因子受体（PDGFR）。总发生率为 5%～60%[1-6]，具体取决于致病药物（表 5-2）。所有级别和高级别不良反应的发生率在瑞戈非尼、索拉非尼和卡博替尼治疗中明显较高。

表 5-2 手足皮肤反应：多激酶血管生成抑制剂报道的发生率比较（荟萃分析）

致病药物	所有级别发生率（%）	高级别发生率（%）	靶 分 子
瑞戈非尼	60.5	20.4	$VEGFR1-3$；$PDGFR\alpha-\beta$；$c-KIT$；RAF；$TIE-2$；RET；$P38MAPK$；$FGFR-1$
卡博替尼	35.3	9.5	$VEGFR2$；MET；RET；KIT；$TIE-2$；$Flt3$
索拉非尼	33.8	8.9	$VEGFR2$、3；$PDGFR\beta$；$c-KIT$；RET；RAF
阿西替尼	29.2	9.6	$VEGFR1-3$；$PDGFR\alpha-\beta$；$c-KIT$
舒尼替尼	18.9	5.5	$VEGFR1-3$；$PDGFR\beta$；$c-KIT$；RET；$Flt3$；$CSF-1R$
帕唑帕尼	4.5	1.8	$VEGFR1-3$；$PDGFR\alpha-\beta$；$c-KIT$；RAF

尽管 HFSR 通常表现为轻至中度皮肤反应（1 级和 2 级），但也可能进展成更严重的情况（3 级），是最有可能导致治疗中断甚至停止治疗的皮肤毒性。此外，虽然 HFSR 不危及生

命,但可导致生活质量下降,并可能严重损害患者的日常生活活动[7]。

既往存在的老茧和其他角化过度区域、不合脚的鞋子以及手足的反复摩擦均为个体化的危险因素。HFSR 是剂量依赖性的,剂量越高越严重。有研究表明,女性患者、亚洲患者、有特异性基因多态性的患者以及接受肾细胞癌治疗的患者往往更容易发生 HFSR[8]。它也可能是临床预后的替代标志[9],但还需要更多的前瞻性数据。

1. 临床表现

无论是由哪种药物引起,HFSR 的临床表现都非常相似[2,9-13],通常在治疗开始后 1～5 周出现。其特征是手掌、足底以及任何摩擦增加的部位容易出现触痛、疼痛、双侧对称性红色和角化过度性病变(图 5-1a～d)。与手掌相比,HFSR 更好发于足底且表现更为严重。皮损主要位于压力/摩擦点和易受创伤部位。它们通常分布于足底承重部位,如足跟、足外侧和跖趾/跖骨皮肤区域。掌部承压面也常常受累,如指尖、大鱼际、指蹼、手指屈面和覆盖在掌指/指骨间关节伸侧的皮肤。

HFSR 通常开始时有前驱症状,表现为刺痛、烧灼感、麻木、感觉迟钝或不耐受触碰,而后在摩擦和受压区域出现界限清晰的疼痛性黄色角化过度的斑块("胼胝样角化过度")。常见皮损周围红色边缘(见图 5-1a～d)。炎症期偶见大的紧张性水疱和肿胀,患者可能难以行走和握物困难;消退期则可见大量脱屑。

值得注意的是,HFSR 与化疗相关的手足综合征明显不同,后者通常表现为掌跖弥漫、对称、有触痛的红斑,可有水疱和溃疡(图 5-1e、f)。

2. 组织病理学表现

在这种情况下进行的组织病理学研究相对较少[11,14]。皮肤活检显示表皮增生伴棘层肥厚、乳头瘤样增生、角化不全、角化不良呈带状散在分布以及角质形成细胞空泡变性,真皮内血管周围轻度的淋巴、组织细胞浸润。角质形成细胞的改变程度与暴露在多激酶血管生成抑制剂的时间有关。

HFSR 的临床表现相当典型,在这种情况下不应当进行皮肤活检。

3. 发病机制

HFSR 确切的发病机制尚未明确,可能是多因素的。然而,HFSR 的发展似乎与多激酶抑制剂的剂量增加相关,这表明可能是直接作用的效应。其他特定的摩擦区域(肘部、瘢痕、掌指关节和指骨间关节伸侧,见图 5-1d)出现类似皮损,提示亚临床型反复的微小创伤可能促进 HFSR 的发生[15]。VEGFR 的抑制,导致内皮细胞的修复机制被破坏,尤其是受压和摩擦部位,可使患者易于发生 HFSR。抑制 VEGFR 可能是必需的,但不足以引起 HFSR;要发生 HFSR,PDGFR 也必须被抑制。例如凡德他尼,它不会抑制 PDGFR,则很少导致 HFSR。反过来,单独抑制 PDGFR 不足以解释 HSFR,如 PDGFR 靶向药甲磺酸伊马替尼不会引起 HFSR。同样,特异性阻断 VEGF 通路的贝伐珠单抗不会引起 HFSR。因此,对 VEGFR 和 PDGFR 的双重抑制可能会阻止血管修复机制,导致对普通损伤产生不恰当的修复反应,从而在反复暴露于亚临床创伤的高摩擦/压力区域(如手掌和足底)诱导 HFSR[11,12,15]。

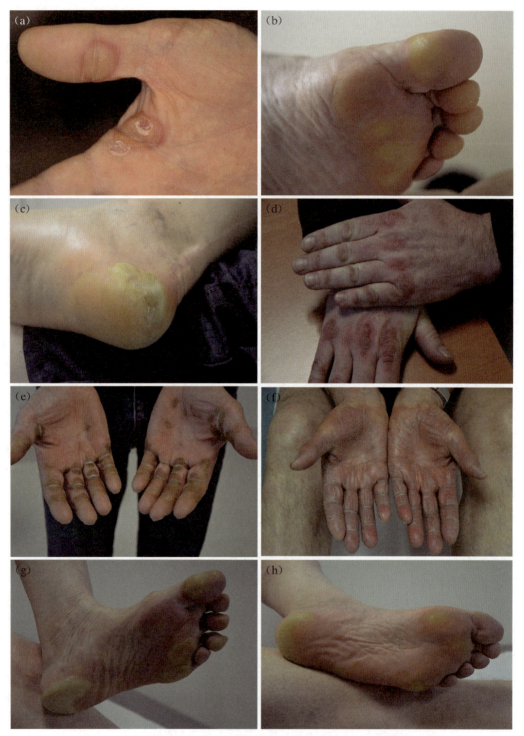

图 5-1 手足皮肤反应,伴有明显的角化过度性病变以及皮损周围的红晕

(a、b)舒尼替尼、(c)瑞戈非尼、(d)卡博替尼治疗在掌指关节和指骨间关节伸侧可见皮损。分别由(e)索拉非尼引起的 3 级 HFSR 和(f)卡培他滨引起的手足综合征。需注意主要的临床区别:(e)角化过度性病变局限于摩擦区域与(f)弥漫性炎症性红斑的比较。BRAF 抑制剂(g)康奈非尼和(h)维罗非尼在足部受压部位引起特征性的胼胝样增厚。

然而,靶向阻断 VEGFR/PDGFR 并不足以解释 HFSR 的所有分子机制,因为选择性 BRAF 抑制剂引起 HFSR 的发生率也很高。据推测,多激酶血管生成抑制剂分泌至外泌汗腺中,导致药物对皮肤的直接毒性。然而,舒尼替尼和索拉非尼经汗液排泄与 HFSR 的发生或严重程度之间没有显著的相关性[1,11]。此外,外泌汗腺中没有明显的组织病理学改变,使得这一理论变得不太可能。

4. 治疗

为了降低 HFSR 的发生率和严重程度,需要进行适当的宣教和咨询,并采取预防措施[8,10,11,13,16]。避免过度受压和反复摩擦是预防 HFSR 的基础。同样重要并需强调的是,HFSR 的发生率和严重程度与剂量的增加密切相关,因此短暂的剂量调整或停药可迅速改善病情。及时识别和处理 HFSR 至关重要,以确保正确的给药剂量、限制剂量调整或停止治疗。

虽然缺乏循证医学建议,治疗主要基于临床经验和专家共识,但已提出一种阶梯式治疗方法(表 5-3)。在治疗的前几周内,必须进行密切监测,要求专业医疗护理人员与患者之间进行密切沟通。

表 5-3 HFSR 的阶梯式治疗方法(美国国家癌症研究所,CTCAE V 4.03)

分级与表现	治疗方法
0级/1级:轻度皮肤改变(如红斑、肿胀或角化过度),不伴疼痛	患者教育和预防措施: • 外用润肤剂,每日 2 次; • 避免创伤性活动、摩擦、过度的压力和揉搓;减少暴露在极端温度下; • 保护易受压或易受摩擦部位; • 使用棉手套和棉袜、凝胶鞋垫、填充鞋垫、减震器、合脚的鞋子;避免过紧的鞋子;识别并预防性去除已有的足底胼胝/角化过度(向足医生就诊和/或局部使用 2%~5% 水杨酸或 10%~50% 尿素软膏)
2级:皮肤改变(如水疱、出血、水肿或角化过度),伴疼痛;日常生活中使用工具受限制	对症处理: • 外用麻醉药(如 2% 利多卡因)和口服止痛药,必要时患处外用高强效类固醇激素(如氯倍他索); • 考虑塞来昔布(100~200 mg/d)或口服类固醇激素 继续使用酪氨酸激酶抑制剂,1~2 周后重新评估并监测严重程度的变化:如果恶化或无法耐受 2 级,则药物剂量减少一个等级,采取预防措施(见 1 级),1~2 周后重新评估;如果改善至 0/1 级,考虑重新增加剂量;如果采取预防措施后皮损恶化或无法耐受 2 级,则对症处理和减少剂量;按 3 级治疗
3级:严重的皮肤改变(如水疱、出血、水肿或角化过度)伴疼痛;日常生活中自理能力受限	对症处理(见 2 级) 停用酪氨酸激酶抑制剂,1 周后重新评估,并监测其严重程度的变化: • 如果症状持续或恶化,则永久停用酪氨酸激酶抑制剂,采取支持性治疗措施; • 如果改善至 0/1 级,采取预防措施(见 1 级),恢复使用酪氨酸激酶抑制剂,但剂量减少一个等级,需密切随访,可考虑重新增加剂量; • 如果采取对症处理、预防性措施和减少剂量后仍无法耐受 2 级或 3 级,则停止治疗

(二) 选择性 BRAF 抑制剂

在接受选择性 BRAF 抑制剂单药(如维罗非尼、达拉非尼)治疗的患者中,20%~60%患者也可观察到类似的症状(图 5-1g、h)[17-20],通常为低级别(3 级<2%)[21-23]。第 2 代 BRAF 抑制剂康奈非尼似乎更容易发生炎症性掌跖角化过度[24]。相反,采用包含 BRAF 和 MEK 抑制剂(如考比替尼、曲美替尼、比美替尼)的联合方案,HFSR 总发生率明显较低(见后"继发性皮肤新生物"节)[19,21-24]。值得注意的是,水疱很少见,足底较少累及。BRAF 相关的 HFSR 可能在整个治疗期间持续存在[25]。

二 诱导性银屑病

(一) 化疗

在使用各种抗增殖化疗药物的患者中,偶然注意到原本存在的银屑病完全或部分缓解[26,27]。相反,多西他赛则有报道出现银屑病皮损加重(图 5-2a、b)[28]。然而,根据我们的经验,紫杉烷类药物可导致银屑病改善或发作。

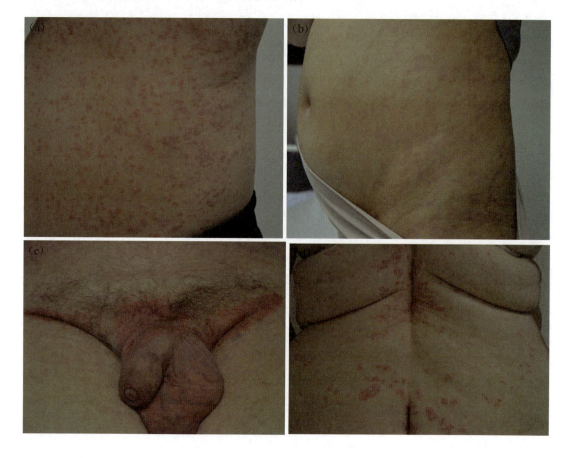

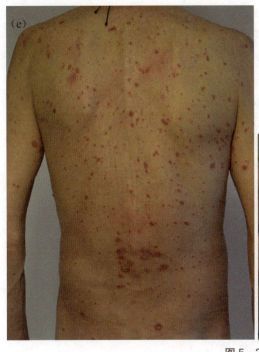
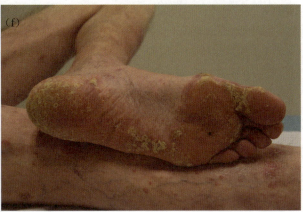

图 5-2 诱导性银屑病

(a)紫杉醇引起的泛发性点滴型银屑病;(b)停止化疗 3 个月后皮损完全消退;(c)伊马替尼引起的反向型银屑病;(d)艾德拉尼引起的斑块型银屑病;(e)抗 PD-1 药物纳武单抗引起的银屑病复发;(f)抗 PD-1 治疗后出现足底皮肤角化伴点滴型银屑病。

(二) 靶向治疗

1. 血管生成抑制剂

通过靶向 VEGF(如贝伐珠单抗)或 VEGFR 1~3(如舒尼替尼、索拉非尼和帕唑帕尼),血管生成抑制剂可改善有银屑病史患者的银屑病斑块[29-32]。此外,给予银屑病小鼠模型外用舒尼替尼软膏,可通过调节角质形成细胞的增殖和凋亡,减轻银屑病样炎症反应[33]。然而,也有报道原有银屑病的患者,在使用贝伐珠单抗和多靶点激酶抑制剂后出现异常的复发或加重[34,35]。

2. EGFR 抑制剂

同样,使用表皮生长因子受体(EGFR)抑制剂(如帕尼单抗、西妥昔单抗、厄洛替尼)治疗,也可以与银屑病的快速和长期改善相关[31,36,37],这可能与直接抑制 EGFR 信号通路有关,后者在银屑病角质形成细胞中过度表达。罕有报道 EGFR 抑制剂诱发银屑病[38]。

3. 抗 CD20 抗体

有个案报道发现,利妥昔单抗可导致慢性斑块型和关节病型银屑病加重或发展,但发病率较低[39-41]。发病机制尚不清楚。有推测 B 细胞缺失可导致 B 细胞介导的 T 细胞调控异常。

4. Bcr-Abl 抑制剂

Bcr-Abl 抑制剂(伊马替尼和较少见于尼洛替尼)也可恶化或促进银屑病(图

5-2c)[42,43]，这可能与调节性 T 细胞下调有关。我们还观察到，血液病患者使用新获批的艾德拉尼和吉瑞替尼（分别靶向 PI3Kδ 和 Flt3）出现斑块型银屑病的严重发作（图 5-2d）。

(三) 抗癌免疫治疗

1. 干扰素

银屑病的新发或加重是聚乙二醇或非聚乙二醇干扰素-α 治疗的明确不良事件，主要表现为斑块型寻常型银屑病。外用治疗往往无效。因此，通常需要中断治疗或系统治疗[44]。

2. 免疫检查点抑制剂

使用抗 PD-1/PD-L1 或抗 CTLA-4 药物发生银屑病的风险也已得到充分证实[45-47]，尽管目前尚不清楚其实际发病率，可以观察到银屑病性关节炎恶化或发生以及更多的银屑病皮疹。斑块状银屑病是最常见的表现，但也有报道点滴型、脓疱型、头皮、掌跖和反向型银屑病（图 5-2e、f）。发病机制尚未明确。已有研究表明，PD-1 信号通路有助于下调 Th1/Th17 信号通路[45]。需要以多学科的方式进行管理。在大多数情况下，免疫治疗可以继续，患者采取外用治疗（如维生素 D 衍生物、外用类固醇激素）进行管理。有时也可采用阿维 A 和 UVB 光疗作为抗肿瘤坏死因子（tumor necrosis factor，TNF）-α 治疗。

三 继发性皮肤新生物

(一) BRAF 抑制剂

1. 概述

作为靶向原癌基因 BRAF 特异性激活突变（V^{600}）的高选择性抑制剂，其主要缺点之一是发生一系列意想不到的皮肤鳞状上皮增殖性病变。其范围从良性的接触性角化过度症、手足皮肤反应（见"手足皮肤反应"节）、Grover 病或毛囊角化病样皮疹，到中间型的疣状角化病，以及恶性的上皮性肿瘤（高分化鳞状细胞癌和角化棘皮瘤）[17-20,25,48-50]。

这些 BRAF 抑制剂引起的角化过度性损害被认为是野生型 BRAF 细胞中 RAS-RAF-MEK-ERK（丝裂原活化蛋白激酶，MAPK）信号通路异常激活的结果，从而引起角质形成细胞增殖增加。有趣的是，与 MEK 抑制剂联合使用（维莫非尼和考比替尼，达拉非尼和曲美替尼，康奈非尼和比美替尼）显著消除了其对鳞状上皮毒性作用的发生率[19,21-25,50,51]。同时抑制 MAPK 信号通路下游的 MEK 抑制剂可阻止这种异常激活，从而减少继发性角化性病变的发生。

值得注意的是，第 2 代 BRAF 抑制剂康奈非尼具有独特的药理学特性，单药治疗很少引起异常的 MAPK 信号通路激活[24]。最后，泛 RAF 抑制剂（如索拉非尼、瑞戈非尼）也可以见到类似的角化性病变，其发生率也较低[12,13]。

2. 疣状角化病

疣状角化病发生在 21%~79% 接受治疗的患者，是使用 BRAF 抑制剂单药最常见的皮肤毒性表现[17-19,21,23,48]。未发现明显的性别差异，但病变在老年患者中更常见。它们在治疗的前 3 个月内逐渐发生，在整个治疗期间持续出现[18,19,25,49]。相反，当患者联合使用

MEK 抑制剂治疗时，疣状角化病则较少发生[19,21,23,25]。

疣状角化病表现为白色、疣状、角化过度的丘疹，直径通常为 2～5 mm[18,19,25,49]。皮损可以在各种解剖位置发生，或者呈广泛分布（曝光和非曝光部位皮肤），或者主要分布在头颈部和躯干，可以看到这类皮损多发（图 5 - 3）[20]。皮肤活检标本显示乳头瘤样增生、棘层肥厚伴角化过度，以及轻至中度的表皮异型[17]。

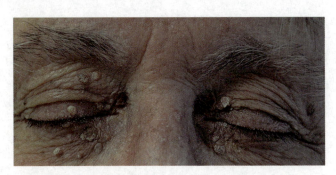

图 5 - 3　BRAF 抑制剂单药治疗出现的多发疣状角化病

由于疣状角化病可以有一定程度的异型性，也可能是鳞状细胞癌的前期病变，建议采取破坏性治疗（如冷冻、电蚀）、外用治疗（如巨大戟醇甲基丁烯酸酯、咪喹莫特）或手术治疗。此外，皮损应定期监测，观察是否有演变为鳞状细胞癌的迹象。病变若体积较大，呈结节状、中央角栓形成，鳞屑性环状边缘或中央溃疡，提示是鳞状细胞癌的临床形态学特征[52]。对任何不典型或可疑的病变，都应进行皮肤活检。

此外，也有报道发生新的脂溢性角化病和角化过度型日光性角化病[17]。

3. 角化棘皮瘤和鳞状细胞癌

根据系列报道，单用维罗非尼/达拉非尼治疗的患者也可能发生高分化鳞状细胞癌（图 5 - 4a～c）和角化棘皮瘤型鳞状细胞癌（图 5 - 5a，b），占 20%～30%[17-22,50,51,53]。康奈非尼单药治疗的发生率则较低[24]。继发性非黑素瘤的皮肤肿瘤，主要发生在治疗的前 3 个月[17,20,49,52-54]，但也会在持续治疗 1 年多后发生 BRAF 诱导的鳞状细胞癌[25]。会阴、生殖器和口腔黏膜也可受累[18,55]。大多数患者通常发生 1～2 个鳞状细胞癌[20]。然而，也有报道发生发疹型鳞状细胞癌[53,56]。

鳞状细胞癌/角化棘皮瘤也可见于使用泛 RAF 抑制剂（如索拉非尼、瑞戈非尼）的患者（图 5 - 5c），但发生率仍明显较低[13,57]。此外，在联合使用 BRAF 和 MEK 抑制剂治疗的患者中，鳞状细胞癌非常罕见，总发生率＜5%[19,21-25,50]。

病变主要位于光损伤皮肤（头面部或四肢），但鳞状细胞癌可发生在各个部位，包括非紫外线暴露部位[17,18,20,49,53,54]。日光性弹性纤维变性和慢性光损伤的程度往往因人而异[20,48,58]。此外，鳞状细胞癌在年长的患者（＞40 岁）以及合并有疣状角化病的患者中更为常见[17,25,49,53]。最后，在抗 BRAF 治疗患者出现的表皮肿瘤（即疣状角化病和鳞状细胞癌）中发现了一种独特的突变谱，容易激活 RAS 突变（主要是 HRAS 亚型），尤其是发生在光损伤部位的病变[20,54,58-60]。据推测，BRAF 抑制剂治疗引起的皮肤鳞状细胞癌是由 MAPK 信号通路的异常增加驱动的，后者是通过在已 RAS 突变的野生型 BRAF 角质形成细胞中形

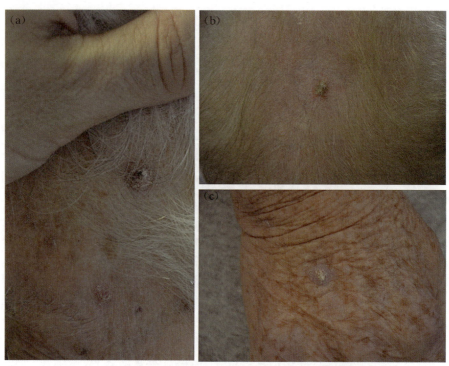

图5-4 (a~c)维罗非尼相关的鳞状细胞癌,发生于慢性光损伤部位

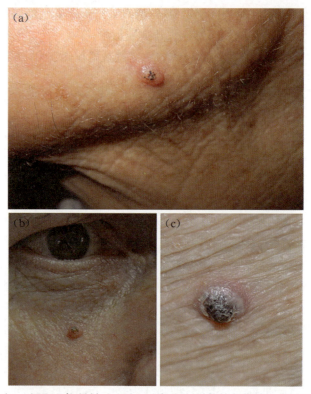

图5-5 (a、b)BRAF抑制剂;(c)泛RAF抑制剂引起的角化棘皮瘤型鳞状细胞癌

成 RAF 同/异二聚体(BRAF – CRAF、CRAF – CRAF)来实现的[54,58,61]。相比之下,同时抑制 MEK 来抑制 MAPK 信号通路的下游,可显著减少皮肤肿瘤的发生[19,21-25,50,51]。此外,其他致癌因素,如高致癌性人乳头瘤病毒和多瘤病毒,在 BRAF 相关的疣状角化病或鳞状细胞癌的发生中不太可能发挥关键作用[17,48,55,56],尽管现有研究数据仍然是相互矛盾的[59,60]。

在这种情况下,肿瘤转移的风险较小。然而,角化棘皮瘤和鳞状细胞癌应手术切除,并留有足够的切缘。对于需要定期或多次手术切除的鳞状细胞癌和疣状角化病患者,提议采用化学预防措施如系统使用维 A 酸类药物[62],外用氟尿嘧啶可能有帮助。仅仅在特殊情况下,才需要剂量调整或停药[20]。关键在于早期发现,患者在整个 BRAF 抑制剂单药治疗期间,需要定期皮肤科随访。

(二) 化疗药物

1. 鳞状细胞癌

现已证实,长期使用抗代谢药物羟基脲治疗可显著增加光分布区域发生日光性角化病或基底细胞癌/鳞状细胞癌的风险[63-65]。此外,经过数月的治疗后,病变可能突然出现,并迅速增长,具有侵袭性[65]。已证实羟基脲会抑制紫外线暴露下角质形成细胞的 DNA 修复。因此,羟基脲可能会干扰表皮基底层的细胞复制。有学者提出"羟基脲相关的鳞状上皮异常增生"这一术语,来区分出羟基脲相关的癌前状态,它会导致更具侵袭性的鳞状细胞癌的发生[65]。建议检查与羟基脲相关的其他角化过度性病变(例如足底/肢端角化病、假性皮肌炎)[64]。

最后,氟达拉滨治疗也可能是皮肤鳞状细胞癌发作和快速生长的触发因素[66]。

2. 炎症性日光性角化病和脂溢性角化病

使用系统性化疗药物后,可使炎症选择性地出现在亚临床型或既往已存在的日光性角化病和脂溢性角化病上。这在氟尿嘧啶及其前体药物卡培他滨(图 5-6)使用中尤其常见,在顺铂、阿糖胞苷、达卡巴嗪、放线菌素 D、多西他赛、多柔比星和长春新碱单独或联合用药中也被观察到[28,67,68]。这可能是化疗对日光性角化病中异常 DNA 合成的直接细胞毒性作用所导致。

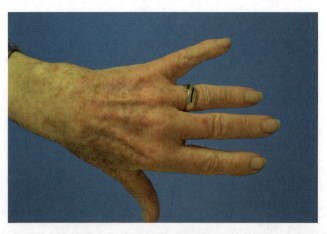

图 5-6 使用卡培他滨患者,在曝光部位出现原有的日光性角化病发生炎症

曝光部位可出现炎症性瘙痒的红色角化鳞屑性丘疹。这种反应通常呈自限性，提示治疗可能有效。建议患者消除疑虑，并提供支持性咨询。如果病变有症状，应予以外用高强效的类固醇激素。

(三) 免疫检查点抑制剂

最近有报道，抗 PD‑1 阻断性治疗患者出现发疹型角化棘皮瘤和炎症性日光性角化病[69]。

(四) 癌症幸存者

癌症幸存者出现继发性肿瘤的总体风险明显更高。非黑色素瘤性皮肤癌是最常见的继发性恶性肿瘤之一，尤其是儿童期接受过治疗的患者或接受异基因造血干细胞移植的患者[70,71]。放疗、长时间的免疫抑制治疗和移植物抗宿主病显然是个体化的风险因素。因此，确保对癌症幸存者进行持续的皮肤科随访，并定期筛查皮肤肿瘤，是至关重要的。

四 毛周角化病和毛发红糠疹样皮疹

(一) Bcr‑Abl 抑制剂

1. 尼洛替尼和达沙替尼

尼洛替尼和达沙替尼是第 2 代 Bcr‑Abl 抑制剂，被批准用于治疗对伊马替尼抵抗（或不耐受）、但表达 Bcr‑Abl 突变的慢性髓系白血病。通过回顾性荟萃分析评估所有级别皮疹的发生率，尼洛替尼和达沙替尼分别约为 34% 和 23%[72]。最常见的表现是瘙痒性毛周角化病样皮疹，可累及额部、面颊、头皮、躯干和四肢近端（图 5‑7a、b）。皮损通常在用药后 2 个月内开始出现，呈剂量依赖性，在停药后消退。类似的病变，包括毛囊周围角化过度性丘疹、角化过度性棘刺和毛囊性红色丘疹，也可见于使用尼洛替尼和达沙替尼者，强烈提示以毛囊为中心的病变过程[72-75]。同样，可以经常见到头皮炎症性非瘢痕性/瘢痕性斑秃伴眉毛受累以及体毛脱落（图 5‑7c）[73,75]。最近有人提出，这些病变使人联想到毛囊扁平苔藓（如 Graham-Little-Piccardi-Lassueur 综合征）[74]。

最突出的组织病理学表现包括毛囊周围纤维化、毛囊内角栓、毛囊萎缩和稀疏的毛囊中心性淋巴细胞浸润[73-75]，发病机制有待阐明。它可能与几种激酶（如 PDGF 受体、RAS/RAF、Src 家族）的直接活性有关，这些激酶可能在表皮稳态中起作用[74,75]。此外，尼洛替尼和达沙替尼可能会减少 TGF‑β 刺激的胶原蛋白产生[72]。

治疗方法包括外用类固醇激素、角质剥脱剂（如乳酸铵、尿素、水杨酸）、抗组胺药（如果需要）。由于瘙痒的不良影响，一些患者可能需要减少剂量或暂时中断治疗。

2. 普纳替尼

普纳替尼是第 3 代 Bcr‑Abl 抑制剂，同时也靶向成纤维细胞生长因子（FGF）、PDGF、VEGF、FMS 样酪氨酸激酶‑3、KIT 和 Src 家族。现已获批用于耐药的慢性髓系白血病和 Ph 阳性的急性淋巴细胞白血病治疗。

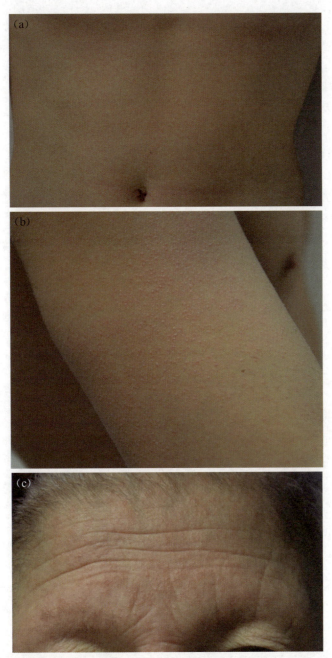

图5-7 (a)达沙替尼引起的弥漫性毛周角化病样皮疹;(b)明显的微小棘刺;(c)尼洛替尼引起的毛囊中心性红色皮疹,伴有特征性2级斑秃(眉毛)

据报道,所有级别的皮疹(除非另有说明)见于约35%接受治疗的患者[74,76]。有时表现为典型的毛发红糠疹样皮疹,在使用普纳替尼2～12周后逐渐出现[77-79]。皮损由界限清晰的粉红-橙色毛囊性丘疹组成,融合成大的瘙痒性斑块伴粉末状鳞屑,可观察到残留的皮岛。病变主要位于躯干、臀部、大腿和腋窝,呈双侧分布。掌跖部位往往不受累。组织病理学特点通常包括角质层增厚,以局灶性角化不全和致密的角化过度交替存在为特征。还可见到真皮浅层少量淋巴细胞浸润、轻度海绵水肿和毛囊周围纤维化[78,79]。治疗依赖于角质剥脱剂、外用类固醇激素、口服/外用维 A 酸或 UVB 治疗,无需中断普纳替尼的治疗。

也有报道,普纳替尼引起板层状鱼鳞病样皮疹[78,80];也可能出现毛囊中心性皮疹,伴明显的角化过度性棘刺和角化不良,类似先前提到的达沙替尼和尼洛替尼[74,78]。最后,患者也可表现为上述皮肤改变的组合。

(二) RAF 抑制剂

在仅接受 BRAF 抑制剂治疗的患者中,也常常观察到弥漫的毛囊中心性红色角化性皮疹,类似毛周角化病的皮疹[18-20,50],>1/3 的患者受到影响[18,50]。病变主要位于躯干和四肢,头部和颈部不受累[18],可伴明显的瘙痒。

使用泛 RAF 抑制剂索拉非尼很少发生类似的皮损,瑞戈非尼更加少见[81]。此外,罕见报道,使用索拉非尼出现毛发红糠疹样皮疹[82]。

五 Grover 病

(一) 概述

Grover 病,即暂时性棘层松解性皮肤病,可发生在各种抗肿瘤治疗中。接受不同化疗方案、放疗、内分泌治疗,或者造血干细胞移植后的患者中有零星报道[83,84]。免疫抑制剂治疗可能是一个支持发病的因素。

皮损主要表现为多形性、瘙痒性红色结痂的丘疱疹,主要位于躯干和上肢。有时皮损可能更加泛发或不典型[83]。组织病理学表现包括表皮棘层松解伴不同程度的角质形成细胞发育不良。

(二) BRAF 抑制剂

Grover 病在选择性 BRAF 抑制剂维罗非尼和达拉非尼单药治疗中更为常见。例如,个案报道在接受达拉非尼治疗的患者中发生率可高达 27%[17]。在临床和组织学上,它与特发性 Grover 病难以鉴别,但病变处有轻度瘙痒[17]。它可以在持续治疗 1 年后出现[25],但在抗 BRAF/MEK 联合治疗中未见报道[19,25]。这可能与正常角质形成细胞中 MAP 激酶通路的异常激活有关(见"继发性皮肤新生物"节)。

(三) 免疫检查点抑制剂

偶有报道使用伊匹单抗和 PD‑1 阻断疗法也会出现 Grover 病[45]。诊断只能通过皮肤活检后得以证实,因此其发病率可能被低估。基底层上棘层松解是孤立存在的(Darier 样形式),真皮内的浸润细胞主要为 $CD4^+$ T 淋巴细胞。尽管皮疹和瘙痒在外用类固醇激素后通常会改善,但在停止治疗后仍可以持续数月。

六 BRAF 抑制剂引起的其他角化过度性反应

(一) 接触性角化过度症

接触性角化过度症仅见于抗 BRAF 治疗的患者。它可以出现在任何慢性摩擦的部位,特别是乳头(图 5-8a)。它还可以影响高达 12% 单药治疗的患者[18,19]。可累及面颊,甚至牙龈和颊黏膜(图 5-8b)[55]。

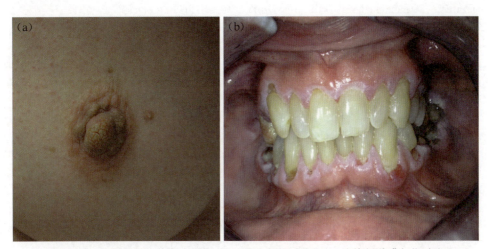

图 5-8　维莫非尼单药治疗后出现(a)乳头角化过度和(b)边缘龈黏膜角化过度

(二) 寻常疣

寻常疣(通常位于手指)的发生,也常见于使用 BRAF 抑制剂后(图 5-9a)[17,19,20,50]。个例可见病毒包涵体和凹空细胞[25]。

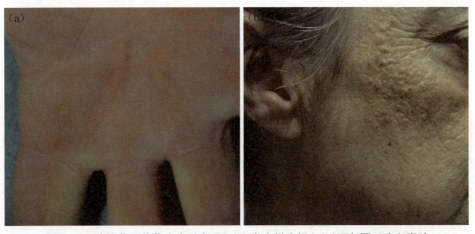

图 5-9　达拉非尼单药治疗后出现(a)寻常疣样皮损和(b)面部粟丘疹和囊肿

(三)囊肿性病变和粟丘疹

使用选择性 BRAF 和泛 RAF 抑制剂治疗的患者可出现表皮样囊肿和粟丘疹(图 5-9b),主要累及面部[12,13,17,18,20,49]。

参考文献

1. Belum VR, Wu S, Lacouture ME. Risk of hand-foot skin reaction with the novel multikinase inhibitor regorafenib: A meta-analysis. *Invest New Drugs* 2013;31:1078-86.
2. Belum VR, Serna-Tamayo C, Wu S, Lacouture ME. Incidence and risk of hand-foot skin reaction with cabozantinib, a novel multikinase inhibitor: A meta-analysis. *Clin Exp Dermatol* 2016;41:8-15.
3. Chu D, Lacouture ME, Weiner E, Wu S. Risk of hand-foot skin reaction with the multitargeted kinase inhibitor sunitinib in patients with renal cell and non-renal cell carcinoma: A meta-analysis. *Clin Genitourin Cancer* 2009;7:11-9.
4. Chu D, Lacouture ME, Fillos T, Wu S. Risk of hand-foot skin reaction with sorafenib: A systematic review and meta-analysis. *Acta Oncol* 2008;47:176-86.
5. Balagula Y, Wu S, Su X, Feldman DR, Lacouture ME. The risk of hand foot skin reaction to pazopanib, a novel multikinase inhibitor: A systematic review of literature and meta-analysis. *Invest New Drugs* 2012;30:1773-81.
6. Fischer A, Wu S, Ho AL, Lacouture ME. The risk of hand-foot skin reaction to axitinib, a novel VEGF inhibitor: A systematic review of literature and meta-analysis. *Invest New Drugs* 2013;31:787-97.
7. Sibaud V et al. HFS-14, a specific quality of life scale developed for patients suffering from hand-foot syndrome. *Oncologist* 2011;16:1469-78.
8. Chanprapaph K, Rutnin S, Vachiramon V. Multikinase inhibitor-induced hand-foot skin reaction: A review of clinical presentation, pathogenesis, and management. *Am J Clin Dermatol* 2016;17:387-402.
9. Wang P, Tan G, Zhu M, Li W, Zhai B, Sun X. Hand-foot skin reaction is a beneficial indicator of sorafenib therapy for patients with hepatocellular carcinoma: A systemic review and meta-analysis. *Expert Rev Gastroenterol Hepatol* 2018;12:1-8.
10. Zuo RC et al. Cutaneous adverse effects associated with the tyrosine-kinase inhibitor cabozantinib. *JAMA Dermatol* 2015;151:170-7.
11. Lacouture ME et al. Evolving strategies for the management of hand-foot skin reaction associated with the multitargeted kinase inhibitors sorafenib and sunitinib. *Oncologist* 2008;13:1001-11.
12. Lee WJ et al. Cutaneous adverse effects in patients treated with the multitargeted kinase inhibitors sorafenib and sunitinib. *Br J Dermatol* 2009;161:1045-51.
13. Robert C, Mateus C, Spatz A, Wechsler J, Escudier B. Dermatologic symptoms associated with the multikinase inhibitor sorafenib. *J Am Acad Dermatol* 2009;60:299-305.
14. Yang CH et al. Hand-foot skin reaction in patients treated with sorafenib: A clinicopathological study of cutaneous manifestations due to multitargeted kinase inhibitor therapy. *Br J Dermatol* 2008;158:592-6.
15. Sibaud V, Delord JP, Chevreau C. Sorafenib-induced hand-foot skin reaction: A Koebner phenomenon? *Target Oncol* 2009;4:307-10.

16. Anderson R, Jatoi A, Robert C, Wood LS, Keating KN, Lacouture ME. Search for evidence-based approaches for the prevention and palliation of hand-foot skin reaction (HFSR) caused by the multikinase inhibitors (MKIs). *Oncologist* 2009;14:291-302.
17. Anforth RM et al. Cutaneous manifestations of dabrafenib (GSK2118436): A selective inhibitor of mutant BRAF in patients with metastatic melanoma. *Br J Dermatol* 2012;167:1153-60.
18. Boussemart L et al. Prospective study of cutaneous side-effects associated with the BRAF inhibitor vemurafenib: A study of 42 patients. *Ann Oncol* 2013;24:1691-7.
19. Carlos G et al. Cutaneous toxic effects of BRAF inhibitors alone and in combination with MEK inhibitors for metastatic melanoma. *JAMA Dermatol* 2015;151:1103-9.
20. Lacouture ME et al. Analysis of dermatologic events in vemurafenib-treated patients with melanoma. *Oncologist* 2013;18:314-22.
21. Robert C et al. Improved overall survival in melanoma with combined dabrafenib and trametinib. *N Engl J Med* 2015;372:30-9.
22. Larkin J et al. Combined vemurafenib and cobimetinib in BRAF-mutated melanoma. *N Engl J Med* 2014;371:1867-76.
23. Long GV et al. Combined BRAF and MEK inhibition versus BRAF inhibition alone in melanoma. *N Engl J Med* 2014;371:1877-88.
24. Dummer R et al. Overall survival in patients with BRAF-mutant melanoma receiving encorafenib plus binimetinib versus vemurafenib or encorafenib (COLUMBUS): A multicentre, open-label, randomised, phase 3 trial. *Lancet Oncol* 2018;19:1315-27.
25. Anforth R, Carlos G, Clements A, Kefford R, Fernandez-Penas P. Cutaneous adverse events in patients treated with BRAF inhibitor-based therapies for metastatic melanoma for longer than 52 weeks. *Br J Dermatol* 2015;172:239-43.
26. Cagiano R et al. Psoriasis disappearance after the first phase of an oncologic treatment: A serendipity case report. *Clin Ter* 2008;159:421-5.
27. Landi D, Santini D, Vincenzi B, La Cesa A, Dianzani C, Tonini G. Dramatic improvement of psoriasis with gemcitabine monotherapy. *Br J Dermatol* 2003;149:1306-7.
28. Sibaud V et al. Dermatological adverse events with taxane chemotherapy. *Eur J Dermatol* 2016;26:427-43.
29. Akman A, Yilmaz E, Mutlu H, Ozdogan M. Complete remission of psoriasis following bevacizumab therapy for colon cancer. *Clin Exp Dermatol* 2009;34:e202-4.
30. Narayanan S, Callis-Duffin K, Batten J, Agarwal N. Improvement of psoriasis during sunitinib therapy for renal cell carcinoma. *Am J Med Sci* 2010;339:580-1.
31. Overbeck TR, Griesinger F. Two cases of psoriasis responding to erlotinib: Time to revisiting inhibition of epidermal growth factor receptor in psoriasis therapy. *Dermatology* 2012;225:179-82.
32. Fournier C, Tisman G. Sorafenib-associated remission of psoriasis in hypernephroma: Case report. *Dermatol Online J* 2010;16:17.
33. Kuang YH et al. Topical sunitinib ointment alleviates psoriasis-like inflammation by inhibiting the proliferation and apoptosis of keratinocytes. *Eur J Pharmacol* 2018;824:57-63.
34. Yiu ZZ, Ali FR, Griffiths CE. Paradoxical exacerbation of chronic plaque psoriasis by sorafenib. *Clin Exp Dermatol* 2016;41:407-9.
35. Du-Thanh A, Girard C, Pageaux GP, Guillot B, Dereure O. Sorafenib-induced annular pustular psoriasis (Milian-Katchoura type). *Eur J Dermatol* 2013;23:900-1.
36. Oyama N, Kaneko F, Togashi A, Yamamoto T. A case of rapid improvement of severe psoriasis during molecular-targeted therapy using an epidermal growth factor receptor tyrosine kinase inhibitor

for metastatic lung adenocarcinoma. *J Am Acad Dermatol* 2012;66: e251-3.
37. Goepel LM, Jacobi A, Augustin M, Radtke MA. Rapid improvement of psoriasis in a patient with lung cancer after treatment with erlotinib. *J Eur Acad Dermatol Venereol* 2018 February 11. doi:10.1111/jdv.14862.
38. Mas-Vidal A, Coto-Segura P, Galache-Osuna C, Santos-Juanes J. Psoriasis induced by cetuximab: A paradoxical adverse effect. *Australas J Dermatol* 2011;52:56-8.
39. Guidelli GM, Fioravanti A, Rubegni P, Feci L. Induced psoriasis after rituximab therapy for rheumatoid arthritis: A case report and review of the literature. *Rheumatol Int* 2013;33:2927-30.
40. Mielke F, Schneider-Obermeyer J, Dörner T. Onset of psoriasis with psoriatic arthropathy during rituximab treatment of non-Hodgkin lymphoma. *Ann Rheum Dis* 2008;67:1056-7.
41. Thomas L et al. Incidence of new-onset and flare of preexisting psoriasis during rituximab therapy for rheumatoid arthritis: Data from the French AIR registry. *J Rheumatol* 2012;39:893-8.
42. Nagai T, Karakawa M, Komine M, Muroi K, Ohtsuki M, Ozawa K. Development of psoriasis in a patient with chronic myelogenous leukaemia during nilotinib treatment. *Eur J Haematol* 2013;91:270-2.
43. Shim JH et al. Exacerbation of psoriasis after imatinib mesylate treatment. *Ann Dermatol* 2016;28:409-11.
44. Afshar M, Martinez AD, Gallo RL, Hata TR. Induction and exacerbation of psoriasis with interferon-alpha therapy for hepatitis C: A review and analysis of 36 cases. *J Eur Acad Dermatol Venereol* 2013;27:771-8.
45. Sibaud V. Dermatologic reactions to immune checkpoint inhibitors: Skin toxicities and immunotherapy. *Am J Clin Dermatol* 2018;19:345-61.
46. Voudouri D et al. Anti-PD1/PDL1 induced psoriasis. *Curr Probl Cancer* 2017;41:407-12.
47. Bonigen J et al. Anti-PD1-induced psoriasis: A study of 21 patients. *J Eur Acad Dermatol Venereol* 2017;31:e254-7.
48. Chu EY et al. Diverse cutaneous side effects associated with BRAF inhibitor therapy: A clinicopathologic study. *J Am Acad Dermatol* 2012;67:1265-72.
49. Sinha R, Edmonds K, Newton-Bishop JA, Gore ME, Larkin J, Fearfield L. Cutaneous adverse events associated with vemurafenib in patients with metastatic melanoma: Practical advice on diagnosis, prevention and management of the main treatment-related skin toxicities. *Br J Dermatol*. 2012;167:987-94.
50. Sanlorenzo M et al. Comparative profile of cutaneous adverse events: BRAF/MEK inhibitor combination therapy versus BRAF monotherapy in melanoma. *J Am Acad Dermatol* 2014;71:1102-9.
51. Ascierto PA et al. Cobimetinib combined with vemurafenib in advanced BRAF V600-mutant melanoma (coBRIM): Updated efficacy results from a randomized, double-blind, phase 3 trial. *Lancet Oncol* 2016;17:1248-60.
52. Belum VR et al. Clinico-morphological features of BRAF inhibition-induced proliferative skin lesions in cancer patients. *Cancer* 2015;121:60-8.
53. Anforth R et al. Factors influencing the development of cutaneous squamous cell carcinoma in patients on BRAF inhibitor therapy. *J Am Acad Dermatol* 2015;72:809-15.
54. Su F et al. RAS mutations in cutaneous squamous-cell carcinomas in patients treated with BRAF inhibitors. *N Engl J Med* 2012;366:207-15.
55. Vigarios E et al. Oral squamous cell carcinoma and hyperkeratotic lesions with BRAF inhibitors. *Br J Dermatol* 2015;172:1680-2.

56. Dika E et al. Human papillomavirus evaluation of vemurafenib-induced skin epithelial tumors: A case series. Br J Dermatol 2015;172:540-2.
57. Arnault JP et al. Keratoacanthomas and squamous cell carcinomas in patients receiving sorafenib. J Clin Oncol 2009;27:e59-61.
58. Oberholzer PA et al. RAS mutations are associated with the development of cutaneous squamous cell tumors in patients treated with RAF inhibitors. J Clin Oncol 2012;30:316-21.
59. Frouin E et al. Cutaneous epithelial tumors induced by vemurafenib involve the MAPK and Pi3KCA pathways but not HPV nor HPyV viral infection. PLoS One 2014;9:e110478.
60. Schrama D et al. Presence of human polyomavirus 6 in mutation-specific BRAF inhibitor-induced epithelial proliferations. JAMA Dermatol 2014;150:1180-6.
61. Ali M, Anforth R, Senetiner F, Carlos G, Fernandez-Penas P. Mechanisms of BRAFi-induced hyperproliferative cutaneous conditions. Exp Dermatol 2016;25:394-5.
62. Anforth R, Blumetti TC, Clements A, Kefford R, Long GV, Fernandez-Peñas P. Systemic retinoids for the chemoprevention of cutaneous squamous cell carcinoma and verrucal keratosis in a cohort of patients on BRAF inhibitors. Br J Dermatol 2013;169:1310-3.
63. Antonioli E et al. Hydroxyurea-related toxicity in 3,411 patients with Ph´-negative MPN. Am J Hematol 2012;87:552-4.
64. Vassallo C et al. Muco-cutaneous changes during long-term therapy with hydroxyurea in chronic myeloid leukaemia. Clin Exp Dermatol 2001;26:141-8.
65. Sanchez-Palacios C, Guitart J. Hydroxyurea-associated squamous dysplasia. J Am Acad Dermatol 2004;51:293-300.
66. Herr D, Borelli S, Kempf W, Trojan A. Fludarabine: Risk factor for aggressive behaviour of squamous cell carcinoma of the skin? Ann Oncol 2005;16:515-6.
67. Peramiquel L, Dalmau J, Puig L, Roé E, Fernández-Figueras MT, Alomar A. Inflammation of actinic keratoses and acral erythrodysesthesia during capecitabine treatment. J Am Acad Dermatol 2006;55:S119-20.
68. Johnson TM, Rapini RP, Duvic M. Inflammation of actinic keratoses from systemic chemotherapy. J Am Acad Dermatol 1987;17:192-7.
69. Freites-Martinez A, Kwong BY, Rieger KE, Coit DG, Colevas AD, Lacouture ME. Eruptive keratoacanthomas associated with pembrolizumab therapy. JAMA Dermatol 2017;153:694-7.
70. Turcotte LM et al. Risk of subsequent neoplasms during the fifth and sixth decades of life in the childhood cancer survivor study cohort. J Clin Oncol 2015;33:3568-75.
71. Leisenring W, Friedman DL, Flowers MED, Schwartz JL, Deeg HJ. Nonmelanoma skin and mucosal cancers after hematopoietic cell transplantation. J Clin Oncol 2006;24:1119-24.
72. Drucker AM, Wu S, Busam KJ, Berman E, Amitay-Laish I, Lacouture ME. Rash with the multitargeted kinase inhibitors nilotinib and dasatinib: Meta-analysis and clinical characterization. Eur J Haematol 2013;90:142-50.
73. Delgado L et al. Adverse cutaneous reactions to the new second-generation tyrosine kinase inhibitors (dasatinib, nilotinib) in chronic myeloid leukemia. J Am Acad Dermatol 2013;69:839-40.
74. Patel AB, Solomon AR, Mauro MJ, Ehst BD. Unique cutaneous reaction to second- and third-generation tyrosine kinase inhibitors for chronic myeloid leukemia. Dermatology 2016;232:122-5.
75. Hansen T, Little AJ, Miller JJ, Ioffreda MD. A case of inflammatory nonscarring alopecia associated with the tyrosine kinase inhibitor nilotinib. JAMA Dermatol 2013;149:330-2.
76. Cortes JE et al. A phase 2 trial of ponatinib in Philadelphia chromosome-positive leukemias. N Engl J Med 2013;369:1783-96.

77. Jack A, Mauro MJ, Ehst BD. Pityriasis rubra pilaris-like eruption associated with the multikinase inhibitor ponatinib. *J Am Acad Dermatol* 2013;69:249-50.
78. Alloo A et al. Ponatinib-induced pityriasiform, folliculocentric and ichthyosiform cutaneous toxicities. *Br J Dermatol* 2015;173:574-7.
79. Eber AE, Rosen A, Oberlin KE, Giubellino A, Romanelli P. Ichthyosiform pityriasis rubra pilaris-like eruption secondary to ponatinib therapy: Case report and literature review. *Drug Saf Case Rep* 2017;4:19.
80. Örenay ÖM, Tamer F, Sarıfakıoğlu E, Yıldırım U. Lamellar ichthyosis-like eruption associated with ponatinib. *Acta Dermatovenerol Alp Pannonica Adriat* 2016;25:59-60.
81. Kong HH, Turner ML. Array of cutaneous adverse effects associated with sorafenib. *J Am Acad Dermatol* 2009;61:360-1.
82. Paz C, Querfeld C, Shea CR. Sorafenib-induced eruption resembling pityriasis rubra pilaris. *J Am Acad Dermatol* 2011;65:452-3.
83. Gantz M, Butler D, Goldberg M, Ryu J, McCalmont T, Shinkai K. Atypical features and systemic associations in extensive cases of Grover disease: A systematic review. *J Am Acad Dermatol* 2017;77:952-7.
84. Villalon G, Martin JM, Monteagudo C, Alonso V, Ramon D, Jorda E. Clinicopathological spectrum of chemotherapy induced Grover's disease. *J Eur Acad Dermatol Venereol* 2007;21:1145-7.

第六章

硬化性皮疹

伯尼斯·邝(Bernice Y. Kwong)

刘孟国 译

在各种抗癌治疗过程中,可发生硬化反应。这些反应很少见,表现形式从局限性皮肤硬化至引起或加重自身免疫性结缔组织病,如系统性硬化症(硬皮病)。此类反应被认为是由于化疗诱导的细胞外基质蛋白积聚到皮肤而致病,可能由 TGF-β 介导。肿瘤治疗引起的硬化反应的临床表现多种多样,包括萎缩性白色带光泽的硬化斑块(硬化性萎缩性苔藓)、皮肤真皮层炎症性硬化和增厚(硬斑病/局限性硬皮病)、下肢硬化呈"倒置香槟瓶"状(脂肪性皮肤硬化症),或疼痛性红色温热斑块,类似蜂窝织炎(假蜂窝织炎)。有系统性硬化症病史的患者可出现病情加重、水肿甚至溃疡。罕见报道某些抗癌药物与新发的自身抗体阳性的系统性硬化症有关。

一 博来霉素所致的肢端硬皮病

抗肿瘤抗生素博来霉素与肺和皮肤的硬化有关[1-3]。皮肤上的硬皮病被认为依赖于累积剂量;有报道称,博来霉素的累积剂量在 51~780 IU。男性可能多见。由于药物通过肾脏排泄,肾功能不全患者可能风险增加[4]。

博来霉素所致的皮肤硬化反应通常累及手和足,呈"肢端硬化"分布,不累及躯干和面部。这种反应始于手、前臂和足部的水肿性斑块,在开始用药后数月出现,随后经数月逐渐演变为手指和关节上的色素性硬化性斑块。手指上的硬化性条带可能妨碍手功能,并导致手指溃疡。在皮肤活检中,可见血管及附属器周围的真皮胶原均质化[2]。虽然通常缺失系统性硬化症的特征,如毛细血管扩张、甲周红斑、皮肤钙质沉着和自身抗体,但皮肤硬化可能合并肺纤维化。

博来霉素所致的硬皮病发病机制尚不清楚,据认为是由于脂质过氧化的直接毒性和 DNA 断裂所致。博来霉素水解酶——负责使博来霉素失活的酶——在皮肤和肺部都缺乏,这与受药物毒性最大的器官相关[5,6]。将博来霉素注射到小鼠皮肤中会导致小鼠硬皮病样皮肤硬化,并伴肺间质化改变;药物在皮肤和肺中浓度较高,可解释这两个器官的局部毒性。受累小鼠硬化部位的皮肤活检显示真皮厚度增加,胶原纤维增厚和沉积,血管壁增厚,肥大细胞增多,前胶原基因表达增加,转化生长因子-β(TGF-β)和趋化因子配体 2(CCL2)表达增加。

博来霉素引起的肢端硬皮病治疗困难,治疗包括硝苯地平、烟酰胺和阿司匹林。在小鼠模型中,贝伐单抗可以预防博来霉素引起的皮肤纤维化[7]。大多数患者停用博来霉素后硬化会得以改善;然而,远端指骨的硬化性改变可持续存在[8]。

二 紫杉烷治疗相关的硬皮病样皮炎

抗微管药物紫杉醇和多西他赛在总累积剂量 $300\sim2\,625\,mg/m^2$[9]时,罕见地出现与之相关的皮肤硬皮病样反应。47%接受紫杉烷治疗的患者出现水肿,在一些病例中,初始的炎症性水肿(图6-1)最终导致硬化和色素沉着,最常见四肢累及,更倾向于下肢。最初的水肿可能在治疗开始后 6 个月至数年内发生,先于硬化出现前 5~12 个月[10,11]。关节受累可能导致挛缩。女性居多,这可能是因为女性乳腺癌和卵巢癌的发病率较高,故使用紫杉烷的频率较高。据报道,紫杉烷治疗引起的硬皮病在单剂量卡铂治疗后会恶化[12]。

虽然紫杉烷引起的肢端硬皮病的临床表现可以模拟系统性硬化症,但通常没有表皮改变或毛细血管扩张,也没有检测到自身抗体。紫杉烷引起的硬皮病,可通过一个独特的临床特点将其与系统性硬化症区分,即该硬化呈近端肢体硬化倾向,而不是更远端的硬化,小腿和脚踝的硬化往往更为明显,使得足末端得以幸免(图6-2)[11]。

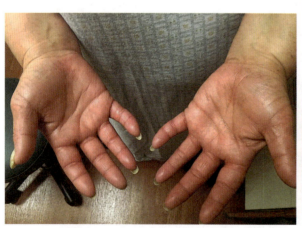

图6-1 接受紫杉烷治疗的患者出现炎症性水肿,导致硬化和色素沉着

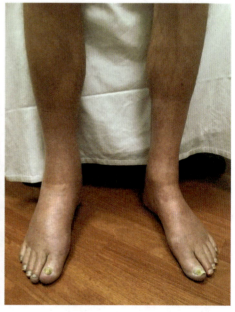

图6-2 接受紫杉烷治疗的患者近端肢体硬化

罕见报道继发于紫杉醇治疗后出现自身免疫抗体阴性的系统性硬化症,伴广泛的硬化和内脏器官受累(包括心肌炎)[13]。罕见报道患者抗核抗体(ANA)阳性,呈离散、斑点型;还有 1 例患者抗着丝点抗体阳性[10]。

在组织病理学检查中,紫杉烷相关性硬皮病患者的皮肤活检结果与系统性硬化症患者相同。病理生理学尚不清楚,可能是激活肿瘤坏死因子-α(TNF-α)、白细胞介素-2(IL-2)、IL-6以及各种细胞因子,刺激成纤维细胞增殖。

紫杉烷引起的硬皮病治疗包括:外用和系统使用类固醇激素、物理疗法和系统使用甲氨蝶呤。一般来说,停药后水肿改善,皮肤最终软化;然而,即使在停药后,皮肤也可能呈持久性"皮包骨样"硬化(图6-3)。

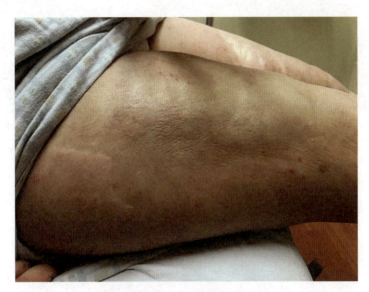

图6-3 持久性"皮包骨样"硬化

三 抗代谢药相关的肢端硬皮病

(一) 5-氟尿嘧啶、卡培他滨、尿嘧啶-替加氟

手足综合征(HFS),又称掌跖感觉丧失性红斑,是5-氟尿嘧啶、其前体药物卡培他滨或尿嘧啶-替加氟(UFT)治疗期间最常见的不良事件,高达68%接受卡培他滨治疗的患者在第2个周期末发生HFS[14]。极少数情况下,患者会出现更严重的硬化型HFS反应,表现为疼痛性、蜡样、有光泽的红斑和水肿,最终硬化、皮肤角化病样增厚,偶尔出现手和手指的肢端硬化(图6-4)[15-18]。在较深色的皮肤类型中,这种硬化型HFS的第1个体征可以是色素沉着(图6-5)[19]。

卡培他滨治疗期间出现硬化性HFS患者的皮肤活检显示,真皮乳头层和网状层硬化,伴有嗜酸性胶原束增厚、均质化,这在经典型HFS中并不常见[15]。治疗包括支持性措施,如外用类固醇激素、润肤、抬高、冷敷和外用麻醉剂。系统使用非甾体抗炎药(如塞来昔布200 mg,每日2次、口服,每个周期14天,用于无心血管病史的患者)可能会有所帮助。在严重情况下,可能需要减少治疗剂量或中断治疗[20]。

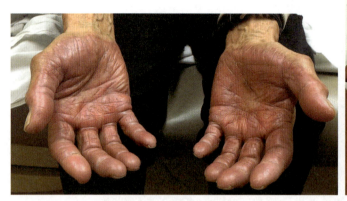
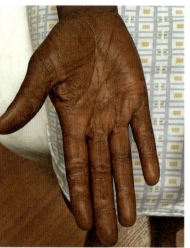

图 6-4　接受 5-氟尿嘧啶治疗的患者出现严重的硬化型 HFS 反应　　图 6-5　接受 5-氟尿嘧啶治疗的患者皮肤呈僵硬、角化病样增厚

(二) 培美曲塞

在使用抗叶酸化合物培美曲塞治疗癌症的过程中，外周水肿很常见，约有 13% 的患者受到影响[21]。与其他抗代谢药物一样，这些患者中的一部分会出现炎症性水肿，随后发展为四肢硬化并伴色素沉着。这种反应又被称为脂肪性皮肤硬化症、"硬化性脂膜炎"或"假蜂窝织炎"。患者最初在四肢出现疼痛性红斑、发热和压痛，代表皮下脂肪的炎症，临床上可能被误为蜂窝织炎（图 6-6），随后出现坚硬、色素沉着并向下束缚的硬化性皮肤，呈"倒置香槟瓶"状。皮肤毒性的严重程度随接受培美曲塞的周期数量增加而增加，并且可能以女性为主。硬皮病样皮疹的皮肤活检显示真皮层增厚伴血管周围淋巴细胞浸润。

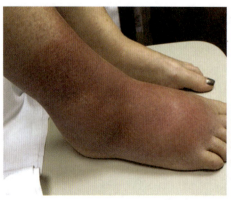
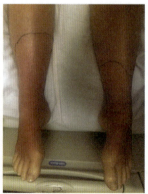

图 6-6　接受培美曲塞治疗的患者出现皮下脂肪炎症

这种反应可能与液体潴留有关，有淋巴水肿、淤滞性皮炎或深静脉血栓并导致下肢水肿病史的患者，其发生风险可能增加。此外，曾接受吉西他滨等其他抗代谢药物治疗的患

者,其发生风险也可能增加。

治疗包括外用类固醇激素、润肤、抬高和治疗水肿的压力袜[22]。系统使用类固醇激素进行预防性治疗(地塞米松 4 mg,每日 2 次,口服;或从治疗前一天开始,每日泼尼松龙 50 mg,连续 3 天),可降低皮肤毒性的严重程度[23]。

(三) 吉西他滨

在使用核苷类似物吉西他滨治疗期间,外周水肿很常见,见于约 20.3% 的患者[24]中。这种皮肤反应称为假蜂窝织炎、脂肪性皮肤硬化样或硬皮病样反应[25]。在这些病例中,炎性水肿表现为疼痛性水肿性红色斑块,通常局限于下肢,开始于踝以上部位,足部不受累。随后,最初的水肿被更多的硬化性皮肤改变所替代,包括"皮包骨样"硬化的皮肤伴色素沉着。可伴有相关的伸展/屈曲困难。临床表现可能被误诊为蜂窝织炎或深静脉血栓形成。

吉西他滨所致的硬化性皮肤改变机制尚不清楚,但理论上认为是继发于药物在皮下脂肪组织的积聚。在开始吉西他滨治疗之前,建议可能存在淤滞性皮炎或淋巴水肿的患者采取预防性干预措施。有系统性硬化症病史的患者接受卡铂和吉西他滨治疗,可增加病变恶化的风险,导致手指坏死[26]。

治疗选择包括:封包条件下外用高强效类固醇激素、抬高、穿紧身衣,或系统使用低剂量类固醇类药物。如果停止用药,皮肤软化通常会随着时间的推移而改善。

(四) 羟基脲

据报道,羟基脲会导致腿部疼痛性水肿,从而引起皮肤木板样硬化,但自身抗体呈阴性。在一病例中,将羟基脲改为阿那格雷后,硬化性病变得以消退[27]。

四 其他药物所致的硬皮病样反应

在没有自身抗体阳性的情况下,硬皮病样皮肤紧绷也有报道见于其他几种化疗药物,包括接受多柔比星和环磷酰胺联合化疗 7 个月至 8 年后的患者出现局限性硬皮病[28]。此外,有报道一卵巢癌患者接受托泊替康第 2 个周期治疗后,手部出现进行性水肿和红斑,随即出现硬化和皮肤紧绷,后来进展为全身皮肤紧绷、手指硬化和小口畸形。ANA 为 1∶640 斑点型;然而,包括抗拓扑异构酶(Scl70)在内的所有其他自身抗体均为阴性,且没有内脏器官累及。托泊替康结合拓扑异构酶可能参与了这种发病机制[46]。1 例接受芳香化酶抑制剂阿那曲唑治疗的乳腺癌患者出现硬化萎缩性苔藓,理论上是由于雌激素水平降低,并外用高强效的糖皮质激素和低剂量的阴道雌激素治疗(插入雌二醇阴道片剂 10 mg,每周 2 次)[29]。

亦有报道,膀胱癌患者膀胱内滴注丝裂霉素 C[30] 和软组织肉瘤患者采用马法兰进行隔离灌注疗法(ILP)[31] 后出现局限性硬皮病。用药物洗脱珠经导管动脉化疗栓塞术(transcatheter arterial chemoem bolization,TACE)治疗肝细胞癌后,可出现皮下脂肪坏死伴硬化[32]。

五 靶向治疗相关的硬化反应

一患者出现与酪氨酸激酶抑制剂舒尼替尼相关的手足疼痛性炎症性水肿，并进展为硬皮病样皮肤和关节肿胀。皮疹在每日服用舒尼替尼 37.5 mg 15 周后发生。自身抗体呈阴性。患者每日服用泼尼松龙 15 mg，每日 2 次外用丙酸倍他米松，每周口服甲氨蝶呤 6 mg 进行治疗。再次给予舒尼替尼后，硬化复发[33]。BRAF 抑制剂维莫非尼也与硬化性改变有关，9.4%接受维莫非尼治疗转移性黑色素瘤患者可出现手掌硬化性结节和挛缩，与掌腱膜挛缩症（Dupuytren 症）样掌跖纤维瘤病一致。这可能发生在治疗后 4～17 个月内[34]。其发病机制尚不清楚，据推测可能是由于 BRAF 野生型细胞（如成纤维细胞）中 MAP 激酶途径的异常活化，或由于 BRAF 被抑制后导致干扰素-γ、CCL4 和 TNF 分泌增加所致。其中 3 例患者在停药后纤维化消退。

六 免疫治疗相关的硬皮病样皮肤反应

皮肤上的免疫相关不良事件（iRAE）在免疫治疗中很常见，此类反应可包括硬化性皮肤反应[35]。据报道，程序性死亡蛋白-1（PD-1）抑制剂帕博利珠单抗与 2 例 BRAF 阳性转移性黑色素瘤患者出现硬皮病样皮肤改变有关。这些患者在第 5 个周期和第 13 个周期后有表现，最初为四肢肿胀和僵硬，随后出现皮肤硬化。即使停止免疫治疗后，该反应仍可能发生和进展。1 例患者伴有雷诺现象和肺部症状，CT 扫描显示肺炎伴磨玻璃样浸润。皮肤活检显示轻度纤维化和硬化，伴有附属器受累和轻微的淋巴细胞炎症。在这些病例中，自身抗体均呈阴性，没有患者具有其他系统性硬化症的特点，如胃肠道症状或甲皱襞毛细血管扩张的表现。治疗选择包括：泼尼松（1 mg/kg，每日 1 次）、静脉注射免疫球蛋白（0.4 mg/kg，每月 5 天）、霉酚酸酯（1 000 mg，每日 2 次）和羟基氯喹（200 mg，每日 2 次）。

接受 PD-1 抑制剂的患者也可能出现硬化性苔藓或硬斑病。纳武单抗与 1 例患者的硬皮病有关，该患者之前曾诊断为硬斑病并缓解了 6 年。在开始使用纳武单抗治疗转移性肺腺癌 2 个月后，出现瘙痒以及有光泽、白色和淡紫色萎缩的圆形斑块[36]。皮肤活检显示硬化性苔藓伴其下方的硬斑病。

七 放疗所致的硬皮病

放疗可导致一些类型的皮肤硬化，这可能很难与皮肤转移性疾病或皮肤感染（如蜂窝织炎）相鉴别。

在急性期，乳房放疗可导致皮下脂肪或筋膜纤维化，称为放射引起的纤维化，通常在治疗后的前 3 个月内迅速发生[37]。

也可能发生延迟性硬化反应。乳腺癌用电离辐射治疗 2～12 年后，可出现硬化萎缩性苔藓[38,39]。皮肤改变，表现为象牙色至白色萎缩性光亮的斑块伴毛细血管扩张，局限于先前放疗的部位，罕见进展到放射区域以外的皮肤。

据报道,1 例外阴鳞状细胞癌患者接受体外放疗(45 Gy,25 次分割照射),随后进行高剂量的阴道袖套近距离放疗(25 Gy,5 次分割照射),治疗一年多后出现硬化萎缩性苔藓[40]。采用 1 类高强效外用类固醇激素治疗有所帮助。

据估计,乳腺癌放疗后,每 1 000 例患者中有 1～2 例(0.2%)发生放疗引起的局限性硬皮病(硬斑病),表现为放疗区域内疼痛性红色硬化性斑块,通常在放疗结束数月至数年后出现[41,42]。最初的炎性斑块,随后变为硬化、色素沉着的斑块。

硬化反应似乎与治疗期间的辐射剂量或急性放射性皮炎无关。其发病机制尚不清楚,但推测是由于辐射诱导产生 Th2 细胞因子,刺激 TGF-β 的产生以及胶原蛋白和其他细胞外基质蛋白的产生。

放射引起的硬化性皮肤反应治疗包括:抗炎药物,如外用、皮损内注射或系统使用类固醇激素;己酮可可碱;超氧化物歧化酶、生育酚(维生素 E)或己酮可可碱-维生素 E 联合进行抗氧化治疗[43]。其他治疗可能包括 UVA-1 治疗[44]、外用钙调磷酸酶抑制剂、甲氨蝶呤或其他免疫抑制药物(包括秋水仙碱、青霉胺),以及体外光化学疗法[45](表 6-1)。

表 6-1 与硬化反应相关的肿瘤治疗方法

药物类别	药物/治疗
烷化剂	卡铂
抗代谢药	卡培他滨 5-氟尿嘧啶 替加氟 培美曲塞 吉西他滨 羟基脲
拓扑异构酶相互作用	托泊替康
抗微管药物	紫杉醇 多西他赛
小分子多激酶抑制剂	舒尼替尼 维莫非尼
免疫治疗	干扰素 纳武单抗 帕博利珠单抗
芳香化酶抑制剂	阿那曲唑
其他	博来霉素 多柔比星 化疗栓塞 放疗 丝裂霉素 C 美法仑

参考文献

1. Finch WR et al. Bleomycin-induced scleroderma. *J Rheumatol* 1980;7:651-9.
2. Cohen IS et al. Cutaneous toxicity of bleomycin therapy. *Arch Dermatol* 1973;107(4):553-5.
3. Kerr LD, Spiera H. Scleroderma in association with the use of bleomycin: A report of 3 cases. *J Rheumatol* 1992;19:294-6.
4. Yamamoto T. Bleomycin and the skin. *Br J Dermatol* 2006;155(5):869-75.
5. Takeda A et al. Immunohistochemical localization of the neutral cysteine protease bleomycin hydrolase in human skin. *Arch Dermatol Res* 1999;291:238-40.
6. Yamamoto T et al. Animal model of sclerotic skin. I: Local injections of bleomycin induce sclerotic skin mimicking scleroderma. *J Invest Dermatol* 1999;112(4):456-62.
7. Koca SS et al. The protective effects of bevacizumab in bleomycin-induced experimental scleroderma. *Adv Clin Exp Med* 2016;25(2):249-53.
8. Kim KH et al. A case of bleomycin-induced scleroderma. *J Korean Med Sci* 1996;11(5):454-6.
9. Battafarano DF et al. Docetaxel (Taxotere) associated scleroderma-like changes of the lower extremities. A report of three cases. *Cancer* 1995;76:110-5.
10. Kawakami T, Tsutsumi Y, Soma Y. Limited cutaneous systemic sclerosis induced by paclitaxel in a patient with breast cancer. *Arch Dermatol* 2009;145(1):97-8.
11. Itoh M et al. Taxane-induced scleroderma. *Br J Dermatol* 2007;156(2):363-7.
12. Konishi Y et al. Scleroderma-like cutaneous lesions induced by paclitaxel and carboplatin for ovarian carcinoma, not a single course of carboplatin, but re-induced and worsened by previously administrated paclitaxel. *J Obstet Gynaecol Res* 2010;36(3):693-6.
13. Winkelmann RR et al. Paclitaxel-induced diffuse cutaneous sclerosis: A case with associated esophagealdysmotility, Raynaud's phenomenon, and myositis. *Int J Dermatol* 2016;55(1):97-100.
14. Capecitabine package insert. https://www.gene.com/download/pdf/xeloda_prescribing.pdf.
15. Trindade F et al. Hand-foot syndrome with sclerodactyly-like changes in a patient treated with capecitabine. *Am J Dermatopathol* 2008;30(2):172-3.
16. Lee SD et al. Hand-foot syndrome with scleroderma-like change induced by the oral capecitabine: A case report. *Korean J Intern Med* 2007;22:109-12.
17. Saif MW et al. Scleroderma in a patient on capecitabine: Is this a variant of hand-foot syndrome? *Cureus* 2016;8(6): e663.
18. Kono T et al. Scleroderma-like reaction induced by uracil-tegafur (UFT), a second-generation anticancer agent. *J Am Acad Dermatol* 2000;42(3):519-20.
19. Narasimhan P et al. Serious hand-and-foot syndrome in black patients treated with capecitabine: Report of 3 cases and review of the literature. *Cutis* 2004;73(2):101-6.
20. Zhang RX et al. Celecoxib can prevent capecitabine-related hand-foot syndrome in stage II and III colorectal cancer patients: Result of a single-center, prospective randomized phase III trial. *Ann Oncol* 2012;23(5):1348-53.
21. Eguia B et al. Skin toxicities compromise prolonged pemetrexed treatment. *J Thorac Oncol* 2011;6(12):2083-9.
22. Shuster M et al. Lipodermatosclerosis secondary to pemetrexed use. *J Thorac Oncol* 2015;10(3): e11-2.
23. Clarke SJ et al. Phase II trial of pemetrexed disodium (ALIMTA, LY231514) in chemotherapy-naïve patients with advanced non-small-cell lung cancer. *Ann Oncol* 2002;13(5):737-41.

24. Aapro MS, Martin C, Hatty S. Gemcitabine: A safety review. *Anticancer Drugs* 1998;9:191-201.
25. Bessis D et al. Gemcitabine-associated scleroderma-like changes of the lower extremities. *J Am Acad Dermatol* 2004;51(2 Suppl): S73-6.
26. Clowse ME, Wigley FM. Digital necrosis related to carboplatin and gemcitabine therapy in systemic sclerosis. *J Rheumatol* 2003;30(6):1341-3.
27. García-Martínez FJ et al. Scleroderma-like syndrome due to hydroxyurea. *Clin Exp Dermatol* 2012;37(7):755-8.
28. Alexandrescu DT, Bhagwati NS, Wiernik PH. Chemotherapy-induced scleroderma: A pleiomorphic syndrome. *Clin Exp Dermatol* 2005;30(2):141-5.
29. Potter JE, Moore KA. Lichen sclerosus in a breast cancer survivor on an aromatase inhibitor: A case report. *J Gen Intern Med* 2013;28(4):592-5.
30. Calistru AM et al. Pseudoscleroderma possibly induced by intravesical instillation of mitomycin C. *J Am Acad Dermatol* 2010;63(6): e116-8.
31. Landau M et al. Reticulate scleroderma after isolated limb perfusion with melphalan. *J Am Acad Dermatol* 1998;39(6):1011-2.
32. Kim HY et al. Supraumbilical subcutaneous fat necrosis after transcatheter arterial chemoembolization with drug-eluting beads: Case report and review of the literature. *Cardiovasc Intervent Radiol* 2013;36(1):276-9.
33. Ohtsuka T. Sunitinib-induced hand-foot syndrome in a renal cell carcinoma: A sclerodermatous and rheumatoid arthritis-like case. *J Dermatol* 2012;39(11):943-4.
34. Vandersleyen V et al. Vemurafenib-associated Dupuytren- and Ledderhose palmoplantar fibromatosis in metastatic melanoma patients. *J Eur Acad Dermatol Venereol* 2016;30(7):1133-5.
35. Barbosa NS et al. Scleroderma induced by pembrolizumab: A case series. *Mayo Clin Proc* 2017;92(7):1158-63.
36. Alegre-Sánchez A et al. Relapse of morphea during Nivolumab therapy for lung adenocarcinoma. *Actas Dermosifiliogr* 2017;108(1):69-70.
37. Rodemann HP, Bamberg M. Cellular basis of radiation-induced fibrosis. *Radiother Oncol* 1995;35(2):83-90.
38. Vujovic O. Lichen sclerosus in a radiated breast. *CMAJ* 2010;182(18): E860.
39. Yates VM, King CM, Dave VK. Lichen sclerosus et atrophicus following radiation therapy. *Arch Dermatol* 1985;121(8):1044-7.
40. Edwards LR et al. Radiation-induced lichen sclerosus of the vulva: First report in the medical literature. *Wien Med Wochenschr* 2017;167(3-4):74-7.
41. Dyer BA, Hodges MG, Mayadev JS. Radiation-induced morphea: An under-recognized complication of breast irradiation. *Clin Breast Cancer* 2016 Aug; 16(4): e141-3.
42. Spalek M, Jonska-Gmyrek J, Gałecki J. Radiation-induced morphea — A literature review. *J Eur Acad Dermatol Venereol* 2015;29(2):197-202.
43. Delanian S, Lefaix JL. Current management for late normal tissue injury: Radiation-induced fibrosis and necrosis. *Semin Radiat Oncol* 2007;17(2):99-107.
44. Kroft EB et al. Ultraviolet A phototherapy for sclerotic skin diseases: A systematic review. *J Am Acad Dermatol* 2008;59(6):1017-30.
45. Fett N, Werth VP. Update on morphea: Part II. Outcome measures and treatment. *J Am Acad Dermatol* 2011;64(2):231-42, quiz 243-4.
46. Ene-Stroescu D, Ellman MH, Peterson CE. Topotecan and the development of scleroderma or a scleroderma-like illness. *Arthritis Rheum* 2002;46(3):844-5.

第七章

手足反应

马修·伯恩鲍姆（Mathew R. Birnbaum），洛伦·佛朗哥（Loren G. Franco），
贝丝·麦克莱伦（Beth N. McLellan）

周丽娟 译

一 手足综合征

（一）流行病学

手足综合征（HFS）于1974年首次被提出，用于描述米托坦治疗后出现的并发症[1]。这种皮疹又被称为掌跖感觉丧失性红斑，最常由细胞毒性化疗药物引起，特别是脂质体多柔比星（PLD）、卡培他滨、多西他赛和5-氟尿嘧啶（5-FU）[2]。HFS的发生率随所应用的单种药物而有所差别，其中PLD和卡培他滨的概率最高，分别为40%～50%和50%～60%（表7-1）[3]。当一些药物联合使用时，例如多柔比星和5-FU连续输注治疗，则发生率明显增高，高达89%[3]。发生HFS的可能性似乎以剂量依赖性的方式增加，因为药物和制剂的半衰期越长，血药浓度则延长，发病率更高。这是导致PLD（半衰期3～4 d）治疗后HFS发生率高于非脂质体多柔比星（半衰期30 h）的一个因素。5-FU持续输注比快速推注发生HFS的概率更高，则进一步支持这种剂量依赖性的关系。同样，5-FU的前体药物如卡培他滨，发生HFS的概率更高，可能是由于它们具有更持久的组织药物浓度[4]。

表7-1 HFS的发生率

	所有级别发生率（%）	高级别发生率（%）
多柔比星+5-FU 持续输注[3]	89	24
脂质体多柔比星（PLD）[3]	40～50	1～20
多柔比星[3,4]	22～29	
卡培他滨[3]	50～60	11～24
多西他赛[3,4]	6～58	
5-氟尿嘧啶[3,4]		
持续输注	34	7
静脉推注	6～13	0.5
阿糖胞苷[3,4]	14～33	

与 HFS 发生相关的其他危险因素包括药物剂量、药物代谢相关的基因变异和女性性别[5]。有趣的是,有研究表明乳腺癌患者中发生 HFS 具有较好的预后[6,7]。一项研究在调查使用贝伐珠单抗和卡培他滨治疗乳腺癌患者时发现,发生 HFS 患者的死亡和疾病进展风险分别降低了 56% 和 44%[7]。需要更多的研究进一步支持这些发现,因为队列间的变量(如中位累积剂量)并不相同。

(二) 发病机制

HFS 的发病机制尚未明确,不同的诱发药物可能具有不同的致病机制[2]。然而,研究表明,药物对角质形成细胞的直接毒性可能是潜在的共同机制。输注后,PLD 首先集中在外泌汗腺的浅部和深部,随后渗透到角质层,在手掌和足底外泌汗腺密度最高处最明显。由于 PLD 的亲水性外层,其似乎更易于通过汗液排泄。最终,PLD 在厚厚的角质层中聚集,引起毒性自由基的释放和氧化损伤[8]。动物模型显示,氧化损伤可能与多柔比星和皮肤中的铜离子相互作用有关,导致活性氧的产生、炎症细胞因子的释放和角质形成细胞的凋亡。研究也确定 IL-8、IL-1β、IL-1α 和 IL-6 是介导趋化因子,可作为治疗的可能靶点[9]。手掌和足底具有更高密度的外泌汗腺导管,再加上这些部位的血管解剖结构、温度梯度以及高的细胞更替时间,有助于解释所观察到的 HFS 掌跖分布,至少在 PLD 的病例中是如此。

不同解剖部位角质形成细胞中酶的变化,可以进一步解释 HFS 的分布。手掌和足底的角质形成细胞显示胸苷磷酸化酶活性增加,该酶负责将前体药物卡培他滨转化为活性的 5-FU[10,11]。小鼠模型显示,卡培他滨和 5-FU 的代谢产物(并非前体分子),通过线粒体和/或离子通道功能障碍引起细胞凋亡[12]。二氢嘧啶脱氢酶(DPD)缺乏者或接受 DPD 抑制剂治疗的患者,发生 HFS 的概率较高,进一步支持 5-FU 代谢产物和 DPD 在 HFS 中的潜在作用[13,14]。

研究还表明,某些基因多态性会增加 HFS 的发生率和严重程度。胞苷脱氨酶(CDD)基因是编码胞苷脱氨酶的基因。胞苷脱氨酶是一种参与嘌呤核苷酸补救合成通路的酶,参与将前体药物卡培他滨转化为 5-FU。CDD 启动子区域的遗传多态性可导致卡培他滨更快地代谢为 5-FU,这与 HFS 的发生率较高有关[15]。同样,与 DNA 合成和叶酸水平相关的基因多态性,如亚甲基四氢叶酸还原酶(MTHFR),也与 HFS 的发生有关[16]。

(三) 临床表现

HFS 通常在开始化疗后 2~21d 内出现[17]。然而,有报道显示,使用某些药物治疗,如口服卡培他滨或持续输注阿糖胞苷,HFS 可晚至 10 个月后发生[3,4,18]。患者常诉掌跖部位感觉障碍,最初是麻刺感,数天内进展为灼痛感。这是由于小的神经纤维损伤导致痛觉和温度觉降低,而轻触觉和本体感觉则不受影响[19]。与神经病变一同发生的是掌跖红斑和水肿,主要见于指/趾的侧面和远端脂肪垫(图 7-1)[20]。日光反应性皮肤分型(Fitzpatrick 皮肤分型)深色的患者也可能出现色素沉着,尤其是在卡培他滨治疗后。在高级别 HFS 中,红斑可进展为脱皮、糜烂和溃疡,也可出现水疱(图 7-2)。有一种独特的紫杉烷特异型 HFS,

被称为关节周围红斑伴甲分离(PATEO)[21]。它表现为大、小鱼际隆起处、关节和跟腱上的红斑(图7-3)。

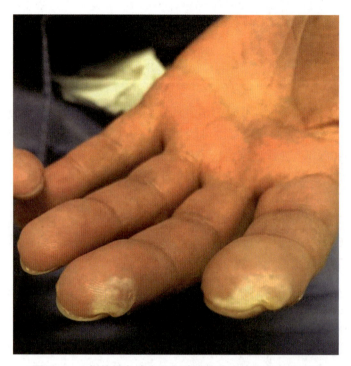

图7-1　1例使用白消安和环磷酰胺治疗的患者出现HFS表现为手掌的红斑和鳞屑(由Eugene Balagula博士提供)。

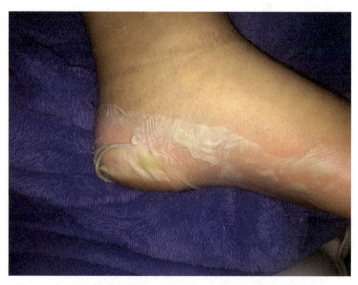

图7-2　使用阿糖胞苷、柔红霉素和依托泊苷治疗的患者出现HFS表现为大疱和脱皮(由Eugene Balagula博士提供)。

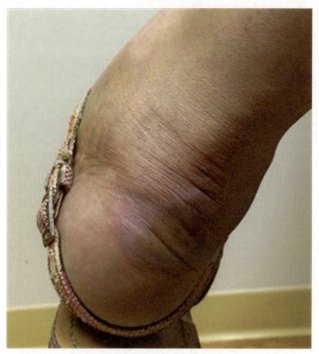

图 7-3　1 例关节周围红斑伴甲分离(PATEO)患者

跟腱上出现的紫色斑块。

(四) 组织病理

虽然 HFS 的组织病理结果没有特异性,但其有类似细胞毒性反应的一系列发现[2]。组织学表现通常与临床严重程度相关。在表皮中观察到的变化,从散在的角质形成细胞坏死伴基底层空泡变性至表皮全层坏死。在真皮中可能存在真皮乳头水肿、血管周围淋巴细胞和嗜酸性粒细胞浸润。也有报道外泌汗腺鳞状汗管化生,与中性粒细胞性外泌汗腺炎表现相似[3,17,22-24]。

(五) 诊断

HFS 是一个临床诊断,鉴别诊断包括接触性皮炎、血管炎、过敏性药疹、多形红斑、红斑肢痛病、肢端博来霉素毒性反应和移植物抗宿主病(GVHD)[5]。感染性病因如皮肤真菌感染,在免疫抑制患者中很常见,因其表现与 HFS 相仿,也应加以鉴别[2,25]。

对 HFS 的严重程度进行分类和分级十分重要,可以帮助皮肤科医生和肿瘤科医生更好地评估和交流患者的临床状态。WHO 和美国国家癌症研究所(NCI)都有 HFS 的分级系统(表 7-2)[4,22]。两种分类法均指出发生 3 级及以上的 HFS 可能要中断治疗、减少药物剂量或停用诱发药物。然而,即使在较常见的轻度 HFS 中,功能损害也可能是非常显著的[5]。HFS-14 等一些经过验证的手段,试图量化 HFS 对患者日常活动的影响[20]。虽然 HFS 不危及生命,通常在停用诱发药物后 1~5 周内消退,但可能会出现一些长期的后遗症。反复发作的 HFS 会引起类似掌跖角化病的表现[10]。有报道一些患者在使用卡培他滨后出现指纹消失,但停药后这些改变似乎恢复正常[26,27]。HFS 也可能增加患者继发感染的风险。极端的案例是 1 例由卡培他滨引起的 HFS 患者继发假单胞菌二重感染导致死亡[10]。

表 7-2 美国国家癌症研究所不良事件的常用术语标准

不良事件	1 级	2 级	3 级	4 级	5 级
掌跖感觉丧失性红斑综合征	轻微的皮肤改变或皮炎(如红斑、水肿或角化过度),无疼痛	皮肤改变(如脱皮、水疱、出血、水肿或角化过度),伴有疼痛;日常生活中使用工具受限	严重的皮肤改变(如脱皮、水疱、出血、水肿或角化过度),伴有疼痛;日常生活中的自理能力受限	—	—

来源:转载自《不良事件通用术语标准(CTCAE)》,4.0 版,2010 年 6 月,美国国立卫生研究院,美国国家癌症研究所。http://evs.nci.nih.gov/ftp1/CTCAE/CTCAE_4.03_2010-06-14_QuickReference_5x7.pdf.可获取全文。2017 年 6 月访问。

(六) 治疗和处理

迄今为止,HFS 最有效的处理是调整剂量或中断药物治疗,症状通常在 1~2 周内改善(表 7-3)[10,23,24]。当 PLD 的治疗每周控制在 10 mg/m², 即使发生 HFS,往往是比较轻微且易于管理的[24,28]。如果患者出现 2 级 HFS,建议延缓治疗,直至症状消退或减轻至 1 级。当发生 3 级或 4 级 HFS 时,建议中断治疗,之后的剂量分别减少 25% 或 50%[24]。尽管已有一些大型研究,但大多数有关 HFS 治疗的文献是病例报告且是没有对照的前瞻性研究。

表 7-3 手足综合征处理建议

级别	症 状	表 现	措施:初次发生	措施:反复发作
1	无或轻度感觉障碍	轻度发红	支持性护理a	支持性护理a
2	感觉障碍但无疼痛	严重发红和/或肿胀	延迟治疗直至症状减轻至 1 级或以下,考虑随后的病程减少剂量	延迟治疗直至症状减轻至 1 级或以下,减少 25% 的治疗剂量
3	感觉障碍伴疼痛	严重发红和/或肿胀	延迟治疗直至症状减轻至 1 级或以下,减少 25% 的治疗剂量	延迟治疗直至症状减轻至 1 级或以下,另外再减少 25% 的治疗剂量
4	疼痛且日常生活活动能力受损	脱皮、水疱、溃疡	延迟治疗直至症状减轻至 1 级或以下,减少 50% 的治疗剂量	停止治疗

来源:来自 von Moos R,等. *Eur J Cancer*, 2008,44(6):781-790. 已经许可使用。
a:支持性护理,即外用保湿乳膏,穿棉袜或戴手套入睡,避免皮肤刺激、极端温度、压力和摩擦。

治疗主要是控制症状,干预措施包括使用高效的外用类固醇激素以减少炎症,对糜烂和溃疡进行伤口护理,外用角质剥脱剂和润肤剂以治疗角化过度,以及使用镇痛剂控制疼痛。一些报道发现,采取预防措施对控制症状可能有好处,包括在给药阶段避免热水浴和剧烈运动[5]。鉴于冷疗和血管收缩剂对预防治疗引起的脱发有益处,这促使在 HFS 中进行类似的研究。通过血管收缩剂限制药物向四肢输送,被认为可使发生 HFS 的风险减轻些。回顾性和前瞻性研究表明,在 PLD 输注期间,使用冰袋或冰水浸泡手足的患者 HFS 发生率较低[3,10,29]。其他研究也表明,在 PLD 治疗期间,对手足使用止汗剂或冰的手套、袜子对减轻 HFS 可能有益[30-32]。遗憾的是,当药物口服或持续输注时,冷疗并不可行[2]。

一项小型的前瞻性研究表明,在发生 2 级及以上 HFS 后,联合口服地塞米松和 PLD 治疗,将来再输注 PLD 时需要减少的剂量可变得很小[33]。吡哆醇(维生素 B_6)最初被认为在 PLD、多西他赛、5-FU 和卡培他滨治疗中可用于预防 HFS[34]。然而,最近的研究包括一项大的荟萃分析发现,在任何化疗中使用吡哆醇均未见获益[21,35,36]。一项随机对照试验发现,在卡培他滨治疗期间使用塞来昔布(每次 200 mg,每日 2 次,持续 14 d),可降低 1 级和 2 级 HFS 的发病率。在使用卡培他滨的情况下,环氧化酶(COX)被认为介导了血管损伤,这解释了为什么使用塞来昔布治疗 HFS 会有效[37]。因此,抑制 COX 可能有助于预防或降低 HFS 的严重程度。

二 手足皮肤反应

一些新型靶向抗癌药物的使用,如多靶点激酶抑制剂(MKI),已表现出其独特的皮肤不良事件特征。这些累及掌跖的皮疹,临床表现与先前描述的 HFS 有所不同;这导致术语手足皮肤反应(HFSR)的应用,将其与更经典的 HFS 相区别[38]。HFSR 与各种药物有关,包括但不限于维莫非尼、瑞戈非尼、卡博替尼、索拉非尼、舒尼替尼、阿希替尼、帕唑帕尼等[39,40]。

(一) 流行病学

所有级别 HFSR 的发生率不一,低至帕唑帕尼治疗的 4.5%,高至瑞戈非尼或维莫非尼治疗的 60%(表 7-4)[39,41,42]。靶向多种激酶的联合疗法与较高的 HFSR 发生率相关。当索拉非尼(一种 MKI)与抗血管内皮生长因子(VEGF)抗体贝伐珠单抗联合使用时,所有级别 HFSR 的发生率高达 79%,高级别反应的发生率达 57%[3]。

表 7-4 手足皮肤反应的发生率

药 物	靶 点	所有级别发生率(%)	高级别发生率(%)
阿昔替尼[64]	VEGFR1~3	29.2	9.6
卡博替尼[65,66]	VEGFR2,c-MET,RET,c-KIT,FLT3,Tie-2	35.3	9.5
达拉非尼	RAF(B)	27[67]	2级:8[67]

(续表)

药　物	靶　点	所有级别发生率(%)	高级别发生率(%)
呋喹替尼	抗VEGFR	64[68]	3级:15[68]
帕唑帕尼[41]	RAF,VEGFR2/3,PGDFR-β,c-KIT,FLT3,RET	4.5	1.8
瑞戈非尼[42]	VEGFR1/2/3,Tie-2,FGFR-1,PDGFR-α/β,c-KIT,RET,RAF,p38 MAPK	60.5	20.4
索拉非尼[69]	VEGFR2/3,PDGFR,RAF(A、B、C),FLT3	59[70]	8.9
索拉非尼+贝伐珠单抗[3]		79	57
舒尼替尼[71]	VEGFR2,PDGFR,c-KIT,FLT3	18.9	5.5
维莫非尼	RAF(B)	25[72]、60[39]	

来源:详见 Lacouture M E, McLellan B N. Hand-foot skin reaction induced by multitargeted tyrosine kinase inhibitors, UpToDate。

注:c-KIT,肥大细胞/干细胞生长因子;FLT3,FMS样酪氨酸激酶-3;MAPK,丝裂原活化蛋白激酶;FDGFR,血小板衍生生长因子受体;RAF,迅速加速纤维肉瘤激酶;RET,转染重排;Tie-2,酪氨酸蛋白激酶受体;VEGFR,血管内皮生长因子受体。

已确定了发生HFSR的一些风险因素。在接受索拉非尼治疗肾细胞癌(RCC)的患者中,与发生2级及以上级别HFSR的相关因素是女性性别、良好的体力状态、较高的治疗前白细胞计数、肺和肝转移,以及多器官受累[43]。

在特定的患者人群中,一些基因多态性与HFSR的发生率增加相关。一项此类研究表明,在接受索拉非尼治疗的韩国肝细胞癌(HCC)患者中,具有VEGF或肿瘤坏死因子-α(TNF-α)单核苷酸多态性的患者HFSR发生率增加[44]。另一项对接受索拉非尼和/或贝伐珠单抗治疗各种实体瘤患者的研究发现,与治疗相关的高血压以及*VEGFR2*、*H472Q*变异等位基因的存在,彼此独立,预示发生HFSR的风险更高[45]。还发现某些恶性肿瘤常与HFSR相关,最显著的是分化型甲状腺癌[46]。

多项研究发现,在使用索拉非尼和舒尼替尼的情况下,患者的生存率与HFSR相关[47-50]。

(二) 发病机制

有证据表明,VEGF受体和血小板衍生生长因子(PDGF)受抑制,导致毛细血管的维持和修复能力不足,至少起了部分作用[2,51,52]。当VEGF和PDGF单独受抑制时,HFSR很少发生。然而,联合治疗同时阻断这两种生长因子时,则HFSR的发生率变得更高(表7-4)[2,3]。

(三) 临床表现

HFSR通常出现在治疗开始的前2～4周内[53]。与HFS相比,HFSR更常累及足底而非手掌。它也易发生于摩擦和压力大的部位，比如趾间趾蹼、足的侧面和其他易受摩擦区域（图7-4）[2,5]。该反应通常表现为红斑基础上局灶性角化过度的胼胝样病变（图7-5）。这与HFS中观察到的更为弥漫、但界限清晰的红斑和鳞屑形成鲜明对比[2]。病变初起可表现为大疱或水疱，常见于足跟、指尖和关节上方（图7-6、图7-7）[52]。HFSR还可引起感觉异常、疼痛、耐热性降低，严重时患者日常生活活动能力受限，例如穿衣打扮[53]。

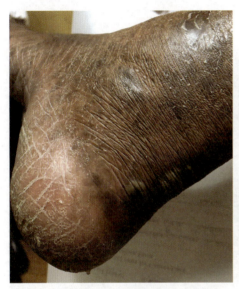

图7-4 1例使用卡博替尼治疗的患者在靴子摩擦区域出现HFSR

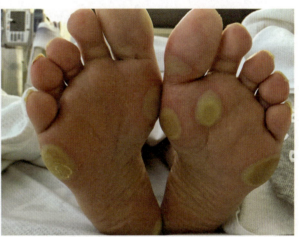

图7-5 1例使用瑞戈非尼治疗的患者出现HFSR

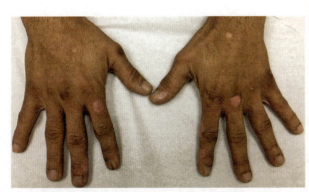

图7-6 1例使用卡博替尼治疗的患者出现HFSR

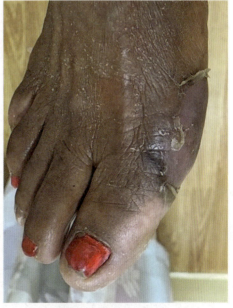

图7-7 1例使用仑伐替尼治疗的患者出现HFSR

(四)诊断

HFSR 是一个临床诊断,应用 NCI 系统可对其严重程度进行分级(表 7-2)[22,24]。应谨记该工具的局限性,因为它不是专门为 HFSR 开发的。此外,该分级可能与患者对皮疹严重程度的感知并不一致[54]。

(五)治疗和处理

最成功的处理方法包括多学科护理,涉及患者、肿瘤科医生、皮肤科医生、足科医生和护士。外用角质剥脱剂可用于所有级别的 HFSR,以治疗观察到的角化过度。10%～40%尿素、6%～12%乳酸铵或 5%～10%水杨酸可局部外用于受累病变,尽量避开皮肤缺损处,以减少可能产生的不适感[52]。检查患者以确定患者的摩擦源或不合身的衣服或鞋子,这对于减少恶化因素至关重要。

对于低级别 HFSR 的疼痛,可外用 2%～6%利多卡因凝胶、乳霜或贴片来治疗。对于 2 级及以上的 HFSR,可系统用药来控制疼痛,包括非甾体抗炎药(NSAID)、阿片类药物或 γ-氨基丁酸(GABA)激动剂[52]。建议使用超强效外用类固醇激素治疗 HFSR 的炎症性红斑区域。小型研究和转化实验发现,外用西地那非[55]、含肝素软膏[56]、含神经酰胺的水胶体敷料[57]和窄带 UVB 光疗[58]也有好处,但仍需更多的研究。

HFSR 处理法则见表 7-5[59]。

表 7-5 手足皮肤反应处理法则

严重度	干 预 措 施
0 级	• 足病医疗咨询 • 保湿剂 • 考虑角质剥脱剂(如每日 3 次使用以尿素为基质的霜剂) • 采取减少压力和摩擦的措施(如穿厚棉袜、合脚的鞋子,避免跑步)
1 级	• 继续上述建议 • 加上外用止痛剂 • 继续当前剂量的抗癌药物,监测严重度变化 • 2 周后重新评估(由医疗专业人员或患者自我报告);若反应恶化或没有改善,进入下一级干预
2 级	• 继续上述建议 • 加上高效的外用类固醇激素(如 0.05%丙酸氯倍他索软膏) • 继续当前剂量的抗癌药物,监测严重度变化 • 2 周后重新评估(由医疗专业人员或患者自我报告);如反应恶化或没有改善,进入下一级干预
3 级或难耐的 2 级	• 继续上述建议及外用药物 • 维持酪氨酸激酶抑制剂(TKI)治疗 7 d 或者直至 HFSR 症状缓解,然后按照每次处方信息恢复较低的剂量 • 如反应恶化或没有改善,有必要根据每次处方信息中断或停止治疗

来源:欲了解更多信息,请参阅 Lacouture M E, McLellan B N 撰写的《多靶点酪氨酸激酶抑制剂诱导的手足皮肤反应》。

预防措施有助于降低发生 HFSR 的风险。在开始使用激酶的靶向治疗前,应先检查患者的手足是否存在角化过度性病变,并由足科医生或皮肤科医生处理。可以建议患者居家操作,例如使用浮石轻柔地去除角质,用温和的润肤剂对手足进行充分的保湿,并注意衣服或鞋子可能存在的摩擦点[52,60]。一项大规模随机对照研究针对刚开始用索拉非尼治疗晚期肝癌的患者,评估每日 3 次预防性外用 10%尿素乳膏对 HFSR 发生率的影响。结果显示,干预组与对照组相比,所有级别和 3 级 HFSR 的发生率较低(所有级别:56% vs.76%;高级别:20.7% vs.29.2%)[61]。然而,该研究具有局限性,比如对照组没有使用任何乳膏,模糊了尿素或润肤剂基质是否与 HFSR 发生率变化相关[62]。另一项近期的回顾性研究发现,预防性口服地塞米松 2 mg 延迟了剂量调整,降低了 3 级 HFSR 的发生率(干预组 3.2% vs.对照组 25.7%)[63]。

三 结语

对 HFS 和 HFSR 的持续研究,有望使临床医生更好地预防和处理这些疾病。随着新型抗肿瘤疗法的出现,掌跖皮肤反应的发生率和临床表现可能会继续进展。未来在基因组学和多态性方面的研究和发现,可能会改变并提高我们对 HFS 和 HFSR 的认识。临床医生将如何利用 HFS 和 HFSR 可能的预后意义来管理和治疗受累患者仍有待确定。

参 考 文 献

1. Zuehlke RL. Erythematous eruption of the palms and soles associated with mitotane therapy. *Dermatologica* 1974;148(2):90-2.
2. Miller KK, Gorcey L, McLellan BN. Chemotherapy-induced hand-foot syndrome and nail changes: A review of clinical presentation, etiology, pathogenesis, and management. *J Am Acad Dermatol* 2014; 71(4):787-94.
3. Degen A et al. The hand-foot-syndrome associated with medical tumor therapy — Classification and management. *J Dtsch Dermatol Ges* 2010;8(9):652-61.
4. Nagore E, Insa A, Sanmartin O. Antineoplastic therapy-induced palmar plantar erythrodysesthesia ("hand-foot") syndrome. Incidence, recognition and management. *Am J Clin Dermatol* 2000;1(4): 225-34.
5. Lipworth AD, Robert C, Zhu AX. Hand-foot syndrome (hand-foot skin reaction, palmar-plantar erythrodysesthesia): Focus on sorafenib and sunitinib. *Oncology* 2009;77(5):257-71.
6. Azuma Y et al. Significant association between hand-foot syndrome and efficacy of capecitabine in patients with metastatic breast cancer. *Biol Pharm Bull* 2012;35(5):717-24.
7. Zielinski C et al. Predictive role of hand-foot syndrome in patients receiving first-line capecitabine plus bevacizumab for HER2-negative metastatic breast cancer. *Br J Cancer* 2016;114(2):163-70.
8. Martschick A et al. The pathogenetic mechanism of anthracycline-induced palmar-plantar erythrodysesthesia. *Anticancer Res* 2009;29(6):2307-13.
9. Yokomichi N et al. Pathogenesis of hand-foot syndrome induced by PEG-modified liposomal doxorubicin. *Hum Cell* 2013;26(1):8-18.
10. Hoesly FJ, Baker SG, Gunawardane ND, Cotliar JA. Capecitabine-induced hand-foot syndrome

complicated by pseudomonal superinfection resulting in bacterial sepsis and death: Case report and review of the literature. *Arch Dermatol* 2011;147(12):1418-23.
11. Milano G et al. Candidate mechanisms for capecitabine-related hand-foot syndrome. *Br J Clin Pharmacol* 2008;66(1):88-95.
12. Chen M et al. The contribution of keratinocytes in capecitabine-stimulated hand-foot-syndrome. *Environ Toxicol Pharmacol* 2017;49:81-8.
13. Kwakman JJM et al. Tolerability of the oral fluoropyrimidine S-1 after hand-foot syndrome-related discontinuation of capecitabine in western cancer patients. *Acta Oncol* 2017;56(7):1023-6.
14. Yen-Revollo JL, Goldberg RM, McLeod HL. Can inhibiting dihydropyrimidine dehydrogenase limit hand-foot syndrome caused by fluoropyrimidines? *Clin Cancer Res* 2008;14(1):8-13.
15. Caronia D et al. A polymorphism in the cytidine deaminase promoter predicts severe capecitabine-induced hand-foot syndrome. *Clin Cancer Res* 2011;17(7):2006-13.
16. Roberto M et al. Evaluation of 5-fluorouracil degradation rate and Pharmacogenetic profiling to predict toxicity following adjuvant Capecitabine. *Eur J Clin Pharmacol* 2017;73(2):157-64.
17. Bolognia JL, Cooper DL, Glusac EJ. Toxic erythema of chemotherapy: A useful clinical term. *J Am Acad Dermatol* 2008;59(3):524-9.
18. Baack BR, Burgdorf WH. Chemotherapy-induced acral erythema. *J Am Acad Dermatol* 1991;24(3):457-61.
19. Stubblefield MD, Custodio CM, Kaufmann P, Dickler MN. Small-fiber neuropathy associated with capecitabine (Xeloda)-induced hand-foot syndrome: A case report. *J Clin Neuromuscul Dis* 2006;7(3):128-32.
20. Sibaud V et al. HFS-14, a specific quality of life scale developed for patients suffering from hand-foot syndrome. *Oncologist* 2011;16(10):1469-78.
21. von Gruenigen V et al. A double-blind, randomized trial of pyridoxine versus placebo for the prevention of pegylated liposomal doxorubicin-related hand-foot syndrome in gynecologic oncology patients. *Cancer* 2010;116(20):4735-43.
22. Common Terminology Criteria for Adverse Events (CTCAE), Version 4.0, June 2010, National Institutes of Health, National Cancer Institute [cited 2017 June 23]. Available from: http://evs.nci.nih.gov/ftp1/CTCAE/CTCAE_4.03_2010-06-14_QuickReference_5x7.pdf.
23. Farr KP, Safwat A. Palmar-plantar erythrodysesthesia associated with chemotherapy and its treatment. *Case Rep Oncol* 2011;4(1):229-35.
24. von Moos R et al. Pegylated liposomal doxorubicin-associated hand-foot syndrome: Recommendations of an international panel of experts. *Eur J Cancer* 2008;44(6):781-90.
25. Wang JZ, Cowley A, McLellan BN. Differentiating hand-foot syndrome from tinea in patients receiving chemotherapy. *Acta Oncol* 2016;55(8):1061-4.
26. van Doorn L, Veelenturf S, Binkhorst L, Bins S, Mathijssen R. Capecitabine and the risk of fingerprint loss. *JAMA Oncology* 2017;3(1):122-3.
27. Wong M, Choo SP, Tan EH. Travel warning with capecitabine. *Ann Oncol* 2009;20(7):1281.
28. Gressett SM, Stanford BL, Hardwicke F. Management of hand-foot syndrome induced by capecitabine. *J Oncol Pharm Pract* 2006;12(3):131-41.
29. Mangili G, Petrone M, Gentile C, De Marzi P, Vigano R, Rabaiotti E. Prevention strategies in palmar-plantar erythrodysesthesia onset: The role of regional cooling. *Gynecol Oncol* 2008;108(2):332-5.
30. Templeton AJ et al. Prevention of palmar-plantar erythrodysesthesia with an antiperspirant in breast cancer patients treated with pegylated liposomal doxorubicin (SAKK 92/08). *Breast* 2014;23(3):

244-9.
31. Scotte F et al. Multicenter study of a frozen glove to prevent docetaxel-induced onycholysis and cutaneous toxicity of the hand. *Am J Clin Oncol* 2005;23(19):4424-9.
32. Scotte F et al. Matched case-control phase 2 study to evaluate the use of a frozen sock to prevent docetaxel-induced onycholysis and cutaneous toxicity of the foot. *Cancer* 2008;112(7):1625-31.
33. Drake RD, Lin WM, King M, Farrar D, Miller DS, Coleman RL. Oral dexamethasone attenuates Doxil-induced palmar-plantar erythrodysesthesias in patients with recurrent gynecologic malignancies. *Gynecol Oncol* 2004;94(2):320-4.
34. Corrie PG et al. A randomised study evaluating the use of pyridoxine to avoid capecitabine dose modifications. *Br J Cancer* 2012;107(4):585-7.
35. Jo SJ, Shin H, Jo S, Kwon O, Myung SK. Prophylactic and therapeutic efficacy of pyridoxine supplements in the management of hand-foot syndrome during chemotherapy: A meta-analysis. *Clin Exp Dermatol* 2015;40(3):260-70.
36. Yap Y et al. Predictors of hand-foot syndrome and pyridoxine for prevention of capecitabine-induced hand-foot syndrome: A randomized clinical trial. *JAMA Oncology* 2017;3(11):1538-45.
37. Zhang RX et al. Celecoxib can prevent capecitabine-related hand-foot syndrome in stage II and III colorectal cancer patients: Result of a single-center, prospective randomized phase III trial. *Ann Oncol* 2012;23(5):1348-53.
38. Porta C, Paglino C, Imarisio I, Bonomi L. Uncovering Pandora's vase: The growing problem of new toxicities from novel anticancer agents. The case of sorafenib and sunitinib. *Clin Exp Med* 2007;7(4):127-34.
39. Boussemart L et al. Prospective study of cutaneous side-effects associated with the BRAF inhibitor vemurafenib: A study of 42 patients. *Ann Oncol* 2013;24(6):1691-7.
40. Massey PR, Okman JS, Wilkerson J, Cowen EW. Tyrosine kinase inhibitors directed against the vascular endothelial growth factor receptor (VEGFR) have distinct cutaneous toxicity profiles: A meta-analysis and review of the literature. *Support Care Cancer* 2015;23(6):1827-35.
41. Balagula Y, Wu S, Su X, Feldman DR, Lacouture ME. The risk of hand foot skin reaction to pazopanib, a novel multikinase inhibitor: A systematic review of literature and meta-analysis. *Investig New Drugs* 2012;30(4):1773-81.
42. Belum V, Wu S, Lacouture ME. Risk of hand-foot skin reaction with the novel multikinase inhibitor regorafenib: A meta-analysis. *Investig New Drugs* 2013;31(4):1078-86.
43. Dranitsaris G, Vincent MD, Yu J, Huang L, Fang F, Lacouture ME. Development and validation of a prediction index for hand-foot skin reaction in cancer patients receiving sorafenib. *Ann Oncol* 2012;23(8):2103-8.
44. Lee JH et al. Genetic predisposition of hand-foot skin reaction after sorafenib therapy in patients with hepatocellular carcinoma. *Cancer* 2013;119(1):136-42.
45. Jain L et al. Hypertension and hand-foot skin reactions related to VEGFR2 genotype and improved clinical outcome following bevacizumab and sorafenib. *J Exp Clin Cancer Res* 2010;29:95.
46. Jean GW, Mani RM, Jaffry A, Khan SA. Toxic effects of sorafenib in patients with differentiated thyroid carcinoma compared with other cancers. *JAMA Oncology* 2016;2(4):529-34.
47. Nagyivanyi K et al. Synergistic survival: A new phenomenon connected to adverse events of first-line sunitinib treatment in advanced renal cell carcinoma. *Clin Genitourin Cancer* 2015;14(4):314-22.
48. Nakano K et al. Hand-foot skin reaction is associated with the clinical outcome in patients with metastatic renal cell carcinoma treated with sorafenib. *Jpn J Clin Oncol* 2013;43(10):1023-9.
49. Poprach A et al. Skin toxicity and efficacy of sunitinib and sorafenib in metastatic renal cell

carcinoma: A national registry-based study. *Ann Oncol* 2012;23(12):3137-43.

50. Lamarca A, Abdel-Rahman O, Salu I, McNamara MG, Valle JW, Hubner RA. Identification of clinical biomarkers for patients with advanced hepatocellular carcinoma receiving sorafenib. *Clin Transl Oncol* 2017;19(3):364-72.

51. Azad NS et al. Hand-foot skin reaction increases with cumulative sorafenib dose and with combination anti-vascular endothelial growth factor therapy. *Clin Cancer Res* 2009;15(4):1411-6.

52. McLellan B, Ciardiello F, Lacouture ME, Segaert S, Van Cutsem E. Regorafenib-associated hand-foot skin reaction: Practical advice on diagnosis, prevention, and management. *Ann Oncol* 2015;26(10):2017-26.

53. McLellan B, Kerr H. Cutaneous toxicities of the multikinase inhibitors sorafenib and sunitinib. *Dermatol Ther* 2011;24(4):396-400.

54. Trotti A, Colevas AD, Setser A, Basch E. Patient-reported outcomes and the evolution of adverse event reporting in oncology. *J Clin Oncol* 2007;25(32):5121-7.

55. Meadows KL et al. Treatment of palmar-plantar erythrodysesthesia (PPE) with topical sildenafil: A pilot study. *Support Care Cancer* 2015;23(5):1311-9.

56. Li JR et al. Efficacy of a protocol including heparin ointment for treatment of multikinase inhibitor-induced hand-foot skin reactions. *Support Care Cancer* 2013;21(3):907-11.

57. Shinohara N et al. A randomized multicenter phase II trial on the efficacy of a hydrocolloid dressing containing ceramide with a low-friction external surface for hand-foot skin reaction caused by sorafenib in patients with renal cell carcinoma. *Ann Oncol* 2014;25(2):472-6.

58. Hung CT, Chiang CP, Wu BY. Sorafenib-induced psoriasis and hand-foot skin reaction responded dramatically to systemic narrowband ultraviolet B phototherapy. *J Dermatol* 2012;39(12):1076-7.

59. Lacouture ME, McLellan BN. *Hand-foot skin reaction induced by multitargeted tyrosine kinase inhibitors*. UpToDate.

60. Manchen E, Robert C, Porta C. Management of tyrosine kinase inhibitor-induced hand-foot skin reaction: Viewpoints from the medical oncologist, dermatologist, and oncology nurse. *J Support Oncol* 2011;9(1):13-23.

61. Ren Z et al. Randomized controlled trial of the prophylactic effect of urea-based cream on sorafenib-associated hand-foot skin reactions in patients with advanced hepatocellular carcinoma. *J Clin Oncol* 2015;33(8):894-900.

62. Negri FV, Porta C. Urea-based cream to prevent sorafenib-induced hand-and-foot skin reaction: Which evidence? *J Clin Oncol* 2015;33(28):3219-20.

63. Fukuoka S et al. Prophylactic use of oral dexamethasone to alleviate fatigue during regorafenib treatment for patients with metastatic colorectal cancer. *Clin Colorectal Cancer* 2017;16(2):e39-44.

64. Fischer A, Wu S, Ho AL, Lacouture ME. The risk of hand-foot skin reaction to axitinib, a novel VEGF inhibitor: A systematic review of literature and meta-analysis. *Investig New Drugs* 2013;31(3):787-97.

65. Belum VR, Serna-Tamayo C, Wu S, Lacouture ME. Incidence and risk of hand-foot skin reaction with cabozantinib, a novel multikinase inhibitor: A meta-analysis. *Clin Exp Dermatol* 2015;41(1):8-15.

66. Zuo RC et al. Cutaneous adverse effects associated with the tyrosine-kinase inhibitor cabozantinib. *JAMA Dermatology* 2015;151(2):170-7.

67. Long GV et al. Dabrafenib and trametinib versus dabrafenib and placebo for Val600 BRAF-mutant melanoma: A multicentre, double-blind, phase 3 randomised controlled trial. *Lancet* 2015;386

(9992):444-51.
68. Xu RH et al. Safety and efficacy of fruquintinib in patients with previously treated metastatic colorectal cancer: A phase Ib study and a randomized double-blind phase II study. *J Hematol Oncol* 2017;10(1):22.
69. Chu D, Lacouture ME, Fillos T, Wu S. Risk of hand-foot skin reaction with sorafenib: A systematic review and meta-analysis. *Acta Oncol* 2008;47(2):176-86.
70. Akaza H et al. A large-scale prospective registration study of the safety and efficacy of sorafenib tosylate in unresectable or metastatic renal cell carcinoma in Japan: Results of over 3200 consecutive cases in post-marketing all-patient surveillance. *Jpn J Clin Oncol* 2015;45(10):953-62.
71. Chu D, Lacouture ME, Weiner E, Wu S. Risk of hand-foot skin reaction with the multitargeted kinase inhibitor sunitinib in patients with renal cell and non-renal cell carcinoma: A meta-analysis. *Clin Genitourin Cancer* 2009;7(1):11-9.
72. Robert C et al. Improved overall survival in melanoma with combined dabrafenib and trametinib. *N Engl J Med* 2015;372(1):30-9.

第八章

抗肿瘤治疗的口腔黏膜反应

艾曼纽尔·维加里奥斯(Emmanuelle Vigarios),文森特·西博(Vincent Sibaud)

杨凡萍 赵 俊 译

一 概述

在抗肿瘤治疗引起的各种毒性反应中,口腔黏膜炎仍然是与细胞毒性化疗和头颈部放疗相关的、主要且常见的不良事件[1]。口腔黏膜炎常给患者带来沉重负担,对生活质量产生负面影响[2,3]。其他化疗或放疗引起的口腔不良事件,如口干、味觉障碍和色素变化,也已得到广泛的认识。

相比之下,新的抗肿瘤治疗(比如靶向治疗和使用免疫检查点抑制剂)引起的口腔不良事件的临床特征仍未得到很好的总结(mTOR抑制剂相关口腔炎除外),且主要以"口腔炎""黏膜炎症""黏膜炎"这些症状描述性疾病进行报道。然而,靶向治疗引起的口腔毒性临床表现具有特异性,与细胞毒性化疗和/或放疗观察到的经典口腔损伤明显不同(表8-1)。此外,超过20%接受治疗的患者出现靶向治疗相关的口腔不良事件,因此靶向治疗相关的口腔不良事件的发病率很高并可能导致永久性的抗肿瘤靶向治疗中断[4]。同样,抗PD-1/PD-L1免疫检查点抗体治疗也可能导致特征性口腔变化[5-7]。

二 细胞毒性化疗药物

(一)黏膜炎症

化疗引起的口腔黏膜炎仍是化疗常见的、剂量依赖性的、可引起严重症状的化疗相关毒性反应[8-20]。20%～40%接受化疗的实体癌患者和大约80%在造血干细胞移植(HSCT)前接受高剂量化疗的患者在化疗的第1个疗程中会经历某种类型的黏膜炎。在随后的化疗周期中,发病率可能会增加到1/3以上,尤其在联合化疗时最为常见。尽管在服用任何形式的细胞毒性化疗药物后都可能发生黏膜炎,但抗代谢药和烷基化剂相关口腔黏膜炎的发生率及其严重程度最高。最常见的相关药物包括甲氨蝶呤、博来霉素、多西他赛、多柔比星、氟尿嘧啶、放线菌素D、长春瑞滨、顺铂、卡铂、伊立替康、环磷酰胺、依托泊苷和紫杉醇。总的来说,血液系统恶性肿瘤接受治疗的患者、20岁以下患者、既往有口腔疾病以及营养状

表 8-1 肿瘤靶向治疗所致的主要口腔改变

靶向治疗药物种类	药物	作用机制/靶点	临床表现	黏膜炎/口腔炎发生率 所有等级（%）	黏膜炎/口腔炎发生率 ≥3级（%）	其他口腔改变	国际非专利名称
mTOR 抑制剂	依维莫司+依西美坦 依维莫司 坦罗莫司	靶向 mTOR 的丝氨酸苏氨酸激酶抑制剂（STKI）[a]	mIAS: mTOR 抑制剂相关的口腔炎（阿弗他溃疡样皮损）非角化性黏膜	62～67 24～64 22～26	8～13 1～9 2～7	味觉障碍 口干	— 飞尼妥（Afinitor®） 特癌适（Torisel®）
EGFR（或 HER1）抑制剂	厄洛替尼 吉非替尼 西妥昔单抗	靶向 EGFR 的酪氨酸激酶抑制剂（TKI）[b] 靶向 EGFR 的单克隆抗体	局限性口腔黏膜炎和阿弗他样皮损 非角化性黏膜	8～20 19～24 7	≤1 ≤1 ≤1 56～72（联合头颈部放疗时）	味觉障碍	特罗凯（Tarceva®） 易瑞沙（Iressa®） 爱必妥（Erbitux®）
HER 抑制剂	帕尼单抗 阿法替尼	靶向 EGF（ErbB1），HER2（ErbB2），ErbB3 以及 ErbB4 受体的 TKI	局限性口腔黏膜炎[c] 和阿弗他样皮损	5 29～64	≤1 3～7	味觉障碍 口干 黏膜出血 和毛细血管扩张	维必施（Vectibix®） 吉泰瑞（Giotrif®）
	达可替尼	靶向 EGFR, HER2 以及 HER4 酪氨酸激酶的不可逆性 TKI		37～41	3～4		尚未上市的拉帕替尼（Tyverb®）
	拉帕替尼	靶向 EGF（ErbB1）以及 HER2（ErbB2）受体的 TKI	非角化性黏膜	6	1		
	曲妥珠单抗	靶向 HER2 的单抗；结合于化疗药物恩美曲妥珠单抗（emtansine）的抗体					赫赛莱（Kadcyla®）

(续表)

靶向治疗药物种类	药物	作用机制/靶点	黏膜炎/口腔炎			其他口腔改变	国际非专利名称
			临床表现	发生率			
				所有等级(%)	≥3级(%)		
血管生成抑制剂	舒尼替尼	靶向 VEGFR 1–3, PDGFR αβ, c–KIT, RET, FLT3, CSF–1R 的 TKI	非特异性口炎	22~27	1~4	良性移行性舌炎 颌骨骨坏死	索坦(Sutent®)
	卡博替尼	靶向 VEGFR, AXL, MET 的 TKI	口腔感觉障碍	22~29	2	味觉障碍 口干症	卡博替尼(Cometriq®)
	索拉非尼	靶向 VEGFR 2–3, PDGFR β, c–KIT, RET, RAF, FLT3 的 TKI	阿弗他样皮损	7~19	0.5~2	色素障碍(sunitinib)	多吉美(Nexavar®)
	帕唑帕尼	靶向 VEGFR 1–3, PDGFR α–β, c–KIT 的 TKI		14	1	良性移行性舌炎 颌骨骨坏死	维全特(Votrient®)
	阿昔替尼	靶向 VEGFR 1–3 的 TKI		15	1	黏膜出血 伤口愈合延迟	英立达(Inlyta®)
	贝伐珠单抗	靶向 VEGF 的单抗					安维汀(Avastin®)

靶向治疗药物种类	药物	作用机制/靶点	主要口腔毒性	国际商品名
BCR–ABL 抑制剂	伊马替尼	靶向 BCR–ABL (Philadelphia 染色体)、PDGFRαβ, c–Kit, CSF–1R, SCF 受体的 TKI	苔藓样反应 "蓝灰色"色素沉着(硬腭) 味觉障碍	格列卫(Glivec®)

（续表）

靶向治疗药物种类	药物	作用机制/靶点	主要口腔毒性	国际商品名
BRAF 抑制剂	达拉非尼 维罗非尼 恩考芬尼（LGX）	靶向 BRAF 的 STKI	黏膜角化过度病变[d]（白线、硬腭、牙龈） 牙龈增生 继发性口腔鳞状细胞癌	泰菲乐（Tafinlar®） 佐博伏（Zelboraf）
ALK 抑制剂	克唑替尼	靶向 ALK、MET、ROS1 的 TKI	味觉障碍	赛可瑞（Xalkori®）
Hedgehog 通路抑制剂	维莫德吉	靶向 SMO 蛋白	味觉障碍，味觉缺失	维莫德吉（Erivedge®）

a：STKI，serine threonine kinase inhibitor，丝氨酸苏氨酸激酶抑制剂；
b：TKI，tyrosine kinase inhibitor，酪氨酸激酶抑制剂；
c：当西妥昔单抗与局部晚期鳞状细胞癌的头颈部放疗联合使用时，常发生严重度等级≥3 级的黏膜炎；
d：当 BRAF 抑制剂与 MEK 抑制剂相关时，这些诱发的病变不会发生；
e：数据未选定的 I 期到 III 期试验（单一疗法药物）获取。
数据来源：Vigarios E, et al. Support Care Cancer, 2017, 25：1713-1739.

况较差者为发病的高风险人群。

尽管黏膜上皮细胞极易受到抑制有丝分裂或干扰DNA合成药物的影响,但口腔黏膜炎并不仅仅是因为这些药物导致了快速分裂的克隆性基底细胞死亡。实际上,正如Sonis最初在一个五步模型[10]中所描述的那样,已经证明化疗会激活黏膜固有层细胞内更复杂的相互作用,包括诱导产生破坏性的活性氧,激活特异转录因子(如NF-κB)和炎症信号通路(如PI3K/Akt、SAPK/JNK、Toll样受体),以及上调促炎症细胞因子(如TNF-α、IL-1β、IL-6)[1-10]。

化疗相关黏膜炎通常在化疗第1个周期后的第4~7天开始。常累及非角化黏膜(口底、软腭、口腔黏膜、舌腹部、嘴唇),角化区域相对较少。先兆期主要表现为红斑和灼烧感。随后可能演变为糜烂和溃疡[1,10,11,13],表面由纤维蛋白、改变了的白细胞和上皮碎片组成的假膜覆盖(图8-1a~d)。初期溃疡的边界清楚,随着病情的进展可能变得广泛、边界模糊和融合。患者常主诉口腔疼痛和口干,常被误认为与食物/液体摄入相关;随后还常出现胃肠道受累症状。

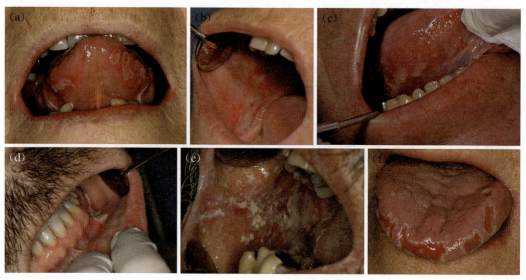

图 8-1 化疗引发口腔黏膜炎

(a)累及舌腹侧的口腔黏膜炎(艾立布林单一疗法);(b)局限性差的溃疡,口腔黏膜上有一层假膜(多西他赛、顺铂和5-氟尿嘧啶联合用药);(c)涉及舌头侧面的黏膜炎(顺铂单一疗法);(d)2级化学性黏膜炎(白消安和环磷酰胺联合用药);(e)HSCT前接受大剂量化疗的患者出现假膜性口腔念珠菌病重叠感染;(f)接受卡培他滨单药治疗的患者出现疱疹性再激活。

多种评估量表可用于对口腔黏膜炎的严重程度进行分级。最常用的是美国国立癌症研究所(NCI)通用毒性标准(CTC,4.0版)和WHO量表[18](表8-2)。

患者发生口腔黏膜炎时常合并口腔真菌感染(口腔念珠菌病;图8-1e)和病毒再激活(疱疹感染;图8-1f)。最后,口腔黏膜损伤可能导致与健康相关的生活质量受损,对患者及其亲属产生不利影响。此外,它可能会增加对系统镇痛药的需求,并延长住院时间。

表8-2 口腔黏膜炎严重度分级

级别	WHO标准	美国国立癌症研究所不良事件通用术语标准(4.0版)
0	无口腔黏膜炎	—
1	红斑和疼痛	无症状或轻微症状；无须干预
2	溃疡；可食固体食物	中度疼痛不影响进食；需要改变饮食习惯
3	溃疡；需要流质饮食(由于口腔黏膜炎)	严重疼痛影响饮食
4	溃疡；无法进食(由于口腔黏膜炎)	产生了危及生命的后果；需要紧急干预
5	——	死亡

最后，化疗引起的口腔黏膜炎应与继发于骨髓抑制的中性粒细胞减少性溃疡相鉴别(图8-2)。临床上，中性粒细胞减少性口腔溃疡常表现为边界清楚的溃疡性病变，周围伴有红斑，在形状、数量和大小上可有所不同，溃疡也可累及角化和非角化黏膜[14]。

一些卫生专业机构报道了口腔黏膜炎的治疗策略。口腔黏膜护理大多采取缓解性治疗措施[15]。《欧洲医学肿瘤学会(ESMO)指南》最终版本的作者重新总结了多国癌症支持治疗协会和国际口

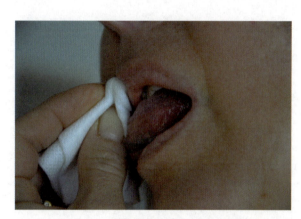

图8-2 中性粒细胞减少性口腔溃疡

腔肿瘤学会(MASCC/ISOO)指南的内容，以进一步促进临床医生的使用[16]。治疗前和治疗期间缓解口腔黏膜损伤的两个关键策略是在整个肿瘤治疗期间维持最佳营养支持，并制定日常口腔卫生常规[17](表8-3)。

表8-3 基础口腔护理、口腔卫生和饮食建议

项目	建议
一般治疗措施	• 每日检查口腔黏膜 • 喝足量的水 • 在肿瘤治疗前进行术前牙齿和牙周筛查，并酌情进行治疗[消除创伤因素(由于牙齿或义齿导致)，牙科感染的治疗] • 治疗期间和治疗后定期进行牙科和牙周检查
牙齿和牙龈护理	• 每日用超软或柔软的牙刷刷牙2~3次，建议使用含低氟无泡沫的牙膏(如果有刺激，请使用无味道的牙膏，例如儿童牙膏/凝胶) • 在进行口腔护理前摘下义齿 • 每餐后用牙线清洁/牙间清洁 • 每日用温和的漱口液漱口4~6次(建议使用无菌水、生理盐水或碳酸氢钠)；在漱口后的前半小时内避免进食和饮水

(续表)

项 目	建 议
	• 清洁可拆卸义齿；如有可能，将义齿浸泡在抗菌溶液中 10 min（若有条件可使用 0.2%氯己定） • 考虑使用口唇保湿剂；注意不应长期在嘴唇上使用凡士林/白石蜡，后者会促进细胞脱水、缺氧，导致口唇继发感染
注意避免	• 含酒精的漱口液和含有十二烷基硫酸钠的牙膏 • 含酒精或过氧化物酶的漱口水产品 • 无相关适应证使用抗真菌或抗菌产品
饮食	• 餐间频繁饮水 • 慢慢咀嚼 • 多样化和清淡的食物 • 使用调味料和调味品进一步增强食品风味，吃冷的食物，避免香味浓郁的食物 • 避免辛辣、酸性、硬、脆和/或高温食物；避免酒精饮料及烟

来源：Vigarios E, et al. Support Care Cancer, 2017, 25: 1713-1739; Lalla R V, et al. Cancer, 2014, 120: 1453-1461。

目前对于化疗相关口腔黏膜炎尚无标准的治疗管理策略，但推荐（基于更高级别的证据）/建议（基于较低级别的证据）[1,16,17]（表 8-4～表 8-7）进行一般对症支持和采取一些防治措施。总的来说，口腔黏膜炎的治疗仍存在挑战。

表 8-4 口腔黏膜炎的预防推荐措施

推荐干预措施	证据等级	治 疗	肿瘤类型
30 min 的口腔冷冻治疗	Ⅱ	接受大剂量 5-氟尿嘧啶化疗的患者	任何肿瘤
光生物调节（低能量激光治疗；波长 650 nm，功率 40 mW，每平方厘米达到 2J/cm² 的剂量）	Ⅱ	接受高剂量化疗条件下行造血干细胞移植（HSCT）的患者，无论是否接受全身照射均适合	任何肿瘤
苄达明漱口水	Ⅰ	接受中等剂量放疗（高达 50 Gy）而不同时接受化疗的患者	头颈肿瘤
KGF-1/帕利夫明（重组人角质形成细胞生长因子-1），剂量为 60 μg/(kg·d)，用于预处理前 3 天，移植后 3 天	Ⅱ	• MASCC/ISOO 原始指南：接受大剂量化疗和全身照射（TBI），然后进行自体干细胞移植的患者 • 更新的 ESMO 指南：接受化疗和/或靶向药物和/或 HSCT 加或不加全身照射（不包括局部至区域放疗）的患者，预计会发展为 3 级或 4 级口腔黏膜炎的患者	血液系统恶性肿瘤

(续表)

不推荐措施	证据等级	治 疗	肿瘤类型
静脉用谷氨酰胺	Ⅱ	为行HSCT接受高剂量化疗(有或无全身照射)的患者	任何肿瘤
艾塞加南抗菌漱口水	Ⅱ	为行HSCT接受高剂量化疗(有或没有全身照射)的患者	任何肿瘤
硫糖铝漱口水	Ⅰ	因癌症进行化疗的患者	任何肿瘤
PTA(多黏菌素B、妥布霉素、两性霉素B)糊剂和BCoG抗菌含片	Ⅱ	进行全身放疗且未同时行化疗的患者	头颈肿瘤
艾塞加南抗菌漱口水	Ⅱ	接受放疗或同时接受放化疗的头颈癌症患者	头颈肿瘤
硫糖铝漱口水	Ⅰ Ⅱ	接受放疗或同时接受放化疗的患者	头颈肿瘤

来源:Peterson D E, et al. Ann Oncol, 2015, 26 (Suppl 5): v139 - v151。
注意:MASCC/ISOO指南中使用的证据级别定义[16,17]如下:
Ⅰ级:从多个精心设计的对照研究荟萃分析中获得的证据;低假阳性和假阴性错误的随机试验(高强度)。
Ⅱ级:从至少一项精心设计的实验研究中获得的证据;具有高假阳性和/或假阴性错误(低强度)的随机试验。
Ⅲ级:从精心设计的准实验研究中获得的证据,如非随机、受控单组、测试前-测试后比较、队列、时间或匹配的病例-对照系列。
Ⅳ级:从精心设计的非实验性研究中获得的证据,如比较和相关描述性研究和案例研究。
Ⅴ级:从病例报告和临床实例中获得的证据。

表8-5 口腔黏膜炎的预防建议

建议措施	证据等级	治 疗	肿瘤类型
口腔护理	Ⅲ	所有肿瘤治疗方式	任何肿瘤
光生物调节(低能量激光治疗;波长约632.8 nm)	Ⅲ	进行放疗且未同时行化疗的患者	头颈肿瘤
口腔冷冻疗法	Ⅲ	为行HSCT接受高剂量美法仑治疗(有或无全身照射)的患者	血液系统恶性肿瘤
补锌剂	Ⅲ	接受放疗或者放化疗的患者	口腔肿瘤
不建议措施	证据等级	治 疗	肿瘤类型
GM-CSF(粒细胞-巨噬细胞集落刺激因子)漱口液	Ⅱ	为自体或者异体干细胞移植接受高剂量化疗的患者	任何肿瘤
系统用毛果芸香碱	Ⅱ Ⅲ	为行HSCT接受高剂量化疗(有或无接受全身照射)的患者 接受放疗的患者	任何肿瘤 头颈肿瘤
氯己定漱口液	Ⅲ	接受放疗的患者	头颈肿瘤
米索前列醇漱口水	Ⅲ	接受放疗的患者	头颈肿瘤

来源与证据级别定义同表8-4的表注。

表8-6 口腔黏膜炎治疗的推荐和建议

推荐干预措施	证据等级	治疗	肿瘤类型
吗啡(患者自控镇痛用)	Ⅱ	进行HSCT的患者	任何肿瘤
不推荐干预措施	证据等级	治疗	肿瘤类型
硫糖铝漱口水	Ⅱ	接受放疗的患者	任何肿瘤
建议干预措施	证据等级	治疗	肿瘤类型
多塞平漱口水(0.5%)(用于控制黏膜炎引起的疼痛)	Ⅳ	所有肿瘤治疗方式	任何肿瘤
芬太尼透皮贴剂(用于控制黏膜炎引起的疼痛)	Ⅲ	接受常规和大剂量化疗的患者,无论是否接受全身照射	任何肿瘤
0.2%吗啡漱口水(用于控制黏膜炎引起的疼痛)	Ⅲ	接受放化疗的患者	头颈肿瘤

来源与证据级别定义同表8-4的表注。

表8-7 抗肿瘤治疗所致口腔黏膜改变的主要干预措施

黏膜改变	主要干预措施
黏膜炎/口腔炎/阿弗他样改变	见表8-3~表8-6,表8-8 讨论:糖皮质激素(局部、病灶内、口服)、吗啡漱口液、全身镇痛剂、光疗 剂量调整(与肿瘤科医生讨论) 放疗疗程的补偿(与放疗师讨论)
口干	基础口腔护理和饮食推荐(见表8-3) 补水、无糖口香糖或糖果兴奋剂;促进唾液分泌:毛果芸香碱、茴三硫片、西维米林、氨甲酰甲胆碱;人工唾液替代品(缓解作用);温热水;经常小口喝水
味觉改变	基础口腔护理和饮食推荐(见表8-3) 剂量调整或药物改变(与肿瘤科医生讨论)
色素改变	无特定的局部治疗措施;为早期发现不典型皮损需定期随访及黏膜病理学活检
口腔苔藓样反应	局部糖皮质激素(如丙酸氯倍他索)治疗疼痛性病变;定期口腔检查并长期随访
口腔感觉障碍	基础口腔护理和饮食推荐(见表8-3) 避免刺激性食物,通过局部止痛药缓解症状 治疗神经病变药物(如氯硝西泮、加巴喷丁、抗抑郁药)
良性游走性舌炎	无特定的局部治疗措施;避免刺激性食物;对于疼痛性病变使用糖皮质激素药物漱口,每日3次,连续使用数天,或外用0.1%他克莫司乳膏
角化过度病变;牙龈增生	无特定的局部治疗措施;为早期发现不典型病变进行每月检查和病理活检
毛细血管扩张/黏膜出血/愈合延迟	基础口腔护理(见表8-3) 药物调整(与肿瘤科医生讨论)

来源:Vigarios E, et al. Support Care Cancer,2017,25:1713-1739。

1. 预防

早期处理措施包括良好的口腔卫生护理。首先,建议进行治疗前口腔筛查,以确诊突发的牙齿或牙周疾病并得到适当的治疗。口腔检查对于消除潜在的创伤来源(不合适的义齿、有缺陷牙的修复、断牙、牙石等)和检测先前存在的黏膜疾病也是必要的[19]。良好的口腔健康还依赖于基本的口腔护理干预[16,17,19](见表8-3)。

报道中有数种药物可用于预防化疗相关口腔黏膜炎,但其疗效并不稳定。口腔冷冻疗法、补锌、低能量激光或系统使用角质形成细胞生长因子——帕利夫明[12,15-17,19]仅用于表8-4和表8-5中报道的特定适应证的推荐或建议治疗方法。以往一些基于低水平研究的个例报道中所描述的其他涂膜剂、抗菌剂或消炎剂不建议采用[1,19]。

2. 治疗

疼痛是口腔黏膜炎最显著的症状,缓解疼痛是长期治疗的基本目标[12,13,15-17,19,20]。一般来说,1级黏膜炎不需要药物干预,良好的口腔护理是需要的,其中包括使用性质温和的漱口水(无菌水、生理盐水或碳酸氢钠)漱口和保持良好的口腔卫生习惯。良好的口腔卫生是缓解口腔黏膜炎症状的关键因素,基本口腔护理方案应被视为降低所有癌症患者口腔黏膜炎疼痛和严重度的一线治疗方案。避免辛辣食物、酒精和吸烟,对于降低口腔黏膜炎的严重度也至关重要(见表8-3)。

对于2/3级黏膜炎,应考虑使用其他的漱口液(如0.2%吗啡漱口液)。还应使用系统镇痛剂或芬太尼透皮贴剂来控制疼痛[1,17]。根据我们的经验,在排除活动性感染后,局部使用糖皮质激素漱口液(例如地塞米松漱口液,0.1 mg/mL)应被视为弥漫性疼痛性黏膜炎的一线治疗。对于可使用局部外用药物治疗的局限性病变,可选择强效糖皮质激素(如0.05%氯倍他索凝胶或乳膏)外用治疗。根据我们的经验,低强度光疗(波长633~685 nm或780~830 nm;功率输出10~150 mW;能量密度2~3 J/cm^2,受治组织表面<6 J/cm^2)[20]与局部糖皮质激素的结合在相隔48 h的2个疗程后,可在一定程度上有效缓解疼痛,并可能促进黏膜炎的愈合。但是,这些结论需要进一步通过前瞻性研究来证实。

高级别口腔黏膜炎的治疗可能需要调整抗肿瘤药物治疗的剂量,以使症状在停止化疗后2周内消失。病变的严重程度和/或复发以及症状恢复所需的时间,将决定是否可以恢复完全给药,或者是否需要减少或停止给药。

最后,严重的黏膜炎会严重影响经口腔营养摄入。应考虑营养师的介入,给予包括与膳食补充剂有关的建议。严重病变有时需要胃造口或鼻胃管喂养[1]。

(二) 色素变化

色素沉着被公认为癌症化疗药物的并发症之一。皮肤(炎症后色素沉着、鞭毛性或网状皮炎、"弥漫性晒黑"、蛇形静脉上色素沉着、发疹性痣等)、指甲(纹状黑甲、横纹黑甲或全黑甲,图8-3a)和口腔黏膜均可能累及。尽管发病机制仍有待确定,但过度色素沉着被认为是继发于化疗药物对黑色素细胞产生直接毒性作用而导致黑色素的过度释放[21,22]。

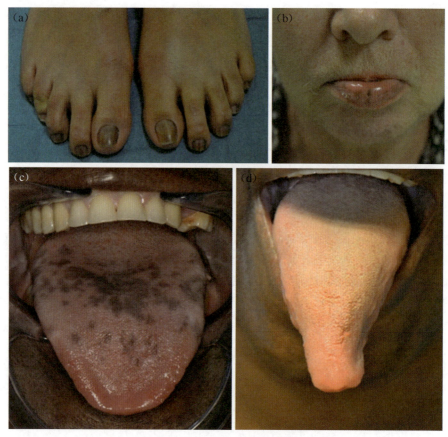

图 8-3 化疗引起的色素变化

(a) 多发性纹状黑甲,累及所有趾甲(羟基脲);(b) 嘴唇上的线状色素沉着斑(卡培他滨);(c) 化疗(卡培他滨)引起的舌背过度色素沉着;(d) 停药 18 个月后同一患者的临床表现,注意病变完全消失。

多种化疗药物[21,22]均可引起口腔黏膜色素变化,尤以白消安、博来霉素、环磷酰胺、顺铂、5-氟尿嘧啶、多柔比星、替加氟、柔红霉素、羟基脲和卡培他滨为多见。由于病变无症状,总体发病率可能仍被低估。黑至褐色的病变可以局部发生,也可以广泛发生,并且可以累及角化和非角化黏膜[嘴唇上的斑片状、线状或弥漫性色素沉着斑(图 8-3b);舌头的腹侧或背侧(图 8-3c)、牙龈、口腔黏膜或腭]。它们可单独存在发展,或与皮肤色素沉着或黑甲同时存在[21,22]。

化疗引起的黏膜色素沉着通常在停药后持续数月,但通常会逐渐消退,有时可完全消失(图 8-3d)。

色素沉着常无特殊的治疗方法,仅需给予患者足够的心理自信,但应该对其作前瞻性随访[21,22]。

(三) 味觉改变

据估计,50%的单纯化疗患者和大约 75%同时接受化疗和头颈部放疗的患者会出现味觉改变[13,23]。化疗类型与发生味觉障碍之间存在统计学上的显著相关性[24]。味觉改变的发生可能是与某些化疗药物(紫杉烷、5-氟尿嘧啶、美法仑、白消安、硫替帕、依托泊苷、环磷酰胺等)或药物组合(R-CHOP、TPF、FEC方案等)有关的不良主诉的首要问题,并可能导致不良的饮食行为[25]。表8-3和表8-7列出了相关治疗干预的建议。

(四) 口干

化疗药物可诱发暂时性(但有时为损伤性)口干症,常表现为口腔灼烧和疼痛。一些患者常先出现口腔金属味,加重味觉障碍[13,14]。它通常在化疗结束后的一年内消失。治疗上首先应提供口腔对症护理(见表8-3、表8-4)。此外,在这种情况下常见牙齿过敏,因此,应每天使用含氟凝胶和牙龈保护层保护牙齿,同时亦可预防龋齿[4]。

(五) 黏膜出血

骨髓抑制可导致自发性或诱发性出血(血小板计数$<20\times10^9/L$)。黏膜出血通常出现在局部创伤后,尤其是在已有牙周病的患者中[13,14]。牙龈出血是最常见的表现。此外,尚可以观察到瘀点、瘀斑或血肿。

三 头颈部放疗

(一) 口腔黏膜炎

几乎所有接受放疗的头颈肿瘤患者都可能发生口腔黏膜炎[1,8,10-12,18,26-28]。病变在最初2~3周以疼痛、充血/红斑形式出现,然后发展为伴有纤维蛋白渗出假膜的溃疡,通常出现在>30 Gy时。病变被严格限制在照射范围内,并可能涉及任何受辐射照射(非角化和角化)的口腔组织(图8-4)。放射性口腔黏膜炎是头颈肿瘤患者最痛苦和致残性的急性毒性反应。口腔疼痛可导致严重的功能损害,严重影响口腔功能和营养摄入。患者也可出现吞咽困难、味觉障碍、口干症和言语困难,所有这些都是发生口腔黏膜炎的原因,并对患者的生活质量产生负面影响。也可能出现脓毒性并发症(单纯疱疹复发、口咽念珠菌病、细菌感染),进一步加重症状并可能诱发全身感染。在任何情况下应该系统地考虑口腔感染,包括不典型或严重的表现,以及超出辐射照射区的黏膜病变外延。

口腔健康和卫生状况差、年龄>65岁、性别(女性风险增加)、伴有牙周病、唾液腺功能障碍、营养状况不佳、肿瘤位置、基因组因素、吸烟、局部创伤和潜在的共病(如糖尿病、肾功能受损)是加重因素。此外,口腔黏膜炎通常在同时接受化疗(如顺铂)和/或靶向治疗(如抗EGFR;参见后文"靶向治疗"中"黏膜炎"节)的头颈部肿瘤患者中更常见、更广泛、更严重。当使用的总辐射剂量增加,以及使用非常规分割放疗时,总发病率较高。三维定向放疗技术和调强放疗(intensity-modulated radiation therapy, IMRT)可以使健康口腔组织对肿瘤周围辐射剂量受到相对保护。

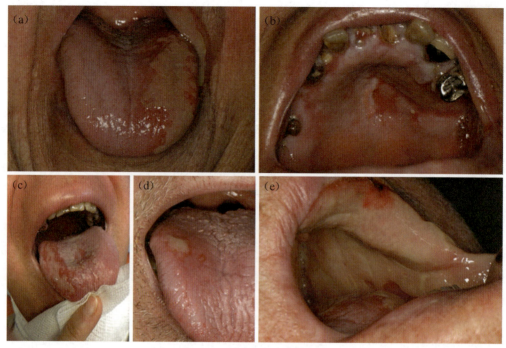

图 8-4 放射诱发的黏膜炎

(a)严重黏膜炎,累及舌背半侧(角化黏膜);(b)边界不清的黏膜炎累及硬腭(角化黏膜);(c)舌头外侧和背侧 3/4 级黏膜炎(角化和非角化黏膜);(d)舌背部局限性损伤(角化黏膜);(e)照射范围内非常广泛的黏膜炎,包括角化和非角化黏膜(颊黏膜、唇黏膜和舌背侧)。

积极的支持性治疗对于这些患者是至关重要的,因为放疗中断或放疗剂量限制可能会通过耐药克隆细胞的重新繁殖,影响局部肿瘤的控制和患者的生存。治疗可能包括使用阿片类镇痛药、胃造瘘管或肠外喂养,有需要时住院治疗。病变是暂时的,通常在停止放疗后 3~8 周内消失。然而,最近发现了持续性或复发性的症状,如慢性萎缩、红斑和/或溃疡[29-31]。

放疗诱导的黏膜炎的处理方法与之前阐述的化疗诱导的黏膜炎相同(见表 8-3、表 8-4)。

(二) 慢性毒性和后遗症

1. 口腔干燥

口干是头颈部放疗后报道的最常见和最显著的口腔毒性[26,32-34]。大唾液腺(腮腺和下颌下腺)和小唾液腺均可发生明显的损害。唾液腺功能减退可导致永久性口干。唾液变得稀少、黏稠。患者也可能经历口腔不适和疼痛。此外,慢性口干可增加口腔感染或龋齿的风险,并可导致说话、咀嚼和吞咽困难,显著影响患者的生活质量。

应系统地提供支持性护理措施(见表 8-3、表 8-4)。治疗主要依赖于用胆碱能激动剂(如毛果芸香碱或西维美林)刺激唾液腺的残余分泌能力。与安慰剂相比,这些药物已被证明能减轻口干症并增加唾液分泌[32-34]。此外,有报道称放疗期间同时给予毛果芸香碱也可增加未受刺激的唾液分泌,可能有短期益处[34]。唾液替代品可能也有用。每日应用局部氟化物凝胶是强制性的,用以限制继发于持续唾液改变的牙齿损害。

最后,需要注意的是,IMRT 可以精确描述肿瘤容积并相对保护有受损风险的器官(如腮腺),与较低的放疗后重度口干症发病率相关[26]。

2. 味觉改变

2/3 接受头颈部放疗的患者味觉发生改变。所有 5 种主要的味觉都会受到影响[23]。辐射可以直接改变嗅觉和味觉,但这些改变也可能与口干症有关。持续的味觉丧失可能是由味觉受体或 C/Aδ 纤维受损以及唾液分泌改变引起的[23,27]。味觉障碍的恢复情况不一,放疗后 2~6 个月可观察到症状改善,但在某些病例中症状可能呈持久性[23]。保留腮腺的 IMRT 可以恢复唾液分泌以及味觉功能[23,26]。处理包括患者宣教和饮食咨询(见表 8-3、表 8-7)。

3. 其他的后遗症

放疗可能导致牙齿和牙周组织的进行性退化,从而增加龋齿和牙周炎的风险。唾液分泌不足也会促进龋齿的发展("辐射性龋齿")[27]。

也可能发生放射后纤维化(包括牙关紧闭)和放射性骨坏死,但这些报道的毒性发生率在当代放疗技术(3D 放疗和 IMRT)下已明显降低[27]。

四 靶向治疗

靶向治疗的口腔毒性可能表现出非常特征性的表现,这与细胞毒性化疗和/或放疗观察到的经典口腔损伤明显不同(见表 8-1)。靶向治疗相关的口腔毒性通常影响 20% 以上的受治患者,并可导致较高的发病率或治疗中断[4,12,16,35-42]。

(一) mTOR 抑制剂

1. mTOR 抑制剂相关口腔炎

(1) 发病率　mTOR 抑制剂相关口腔炎(mTOR inhibitor-associated stomatitis, mIAS)是一种频发且有特征性的口腔毒性。荟萃分析表明,任何级别 mIAS 的总发病率和高级别(≥3 级,NCI - CTCae V4.02)mIAS 的发病率范围分别是 33.5%~52.9% 及 4.1%~5.4%,不管 mTOR 抑制剂的治疗类型(依维莫司、西罗莫司)[44,45,49](见表 8-1)。mIAS 最常发生在第 1 个治疗周期内[44-46],被认为是类效应。mIAS 是与 mTOR 治疗相关的最多发的不良事件,也是最常见的剂量限制性毒性[4,44]。此外,依维莫司联合内分泌药物(依西美坦)治疗乳腺癌与所有级别 mIAS 的发病率增加显著相关[47],有超过 2/3 的受治患者受到影响。

(2) 临床表现　mIAS 的特征是单发或多发、疼痛、边界清楚的圆形/卵圆形浅表性溃疡(口腔炎样),主要发生在非角化黏膜区[4,35,38,43,44,48,49]。病灶直径一般为几毫米,中央灰色区域被病灶外周的红斑晕包围,类似复发性阿弗他溃疡或疱疹性病变(图 8-5)。与化疗诱导的黏膜炎不同,mIAS 通常不累及其他黏膜。

(3) 处理　预防性处理包括促进良好的口腔卫生,依靠基本的口腔护理建议(见

表8-3)。建议在治疗前进行口腔筛查,以确定创伤和牙齿或牙周病暴发的潜在来源。最近第二阶段预防试验(SWISH 试验)[50]、预防性使用地塞米松漱口水(0.5 mg/5 mL,每日 4 次,持续 8 周)在接受依维莫司(10 mg)和依西美坦(25 mg)治疗的晚期或转移性乳腺癌患者的全级别 mIAS 的发病率显著降低(全级别发病率 21.2%,≥2 级发病率<3%,无 3 级发生;间接比较)。

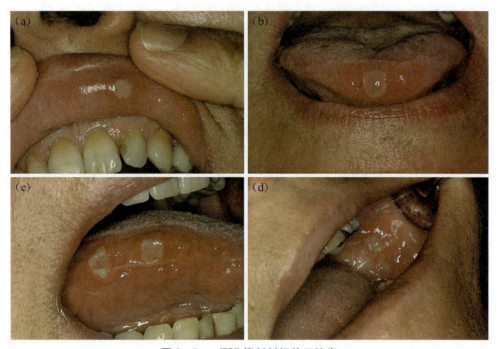

图 8-5 mTOR 抑制剂相关口腔炎

(a、b)依维莫司诱导的典型 mIAS,伴有红晕(病变仅累及非角化黏膜);(c、d)依维莫司和依西美坦联合治疗的患者出现多发性阿弗他溃疡样病变。

根据最新的 ESMO 临床实践指南[16],建议将糖皮质激素作为 mIAS 的一线治疗药物:主要是局部糖皮质激素[糖皮质激素漱口水(如地塞米松漱口水,0.1 mg/mL)或局部应用强效糖皮质激素(0.05%氯倍他索凝胶或乳膏)],如有需要,可使用病灶内或系统糖皮质激素治疗。根据我们的经验,这种"激素疗法"可以与光生物调节疗法联合(低能量激光治疗:波长 633~685 nm 或 780~830 nm;功率输出为 10~150 mW;能量密度在组织表面 2~3 J/cm² 且≤6 J/cm²)[4]。高级别 mIAS 也可以通过剂量调整来处理(表 8-8)。例如,在主要的临床试验中,大约 5% 和 2% 的治疗患者需要修改剂量和停止治疗[44,46,48,49]。病变的严重程度和/或复发,以及恢复所需的时间,将决定是否可以恢复完全剂量,或是否需要减量或停药[4,39,47]。

表 8-8　mIAS 的改进管理流程

1 级[a] (黏膜红斑,无症状或轻微症状)	2 级 (斑片状溃疡伴中度疼痛;不影响口服)	3 级 (融合性溃疡或假膜,伴剧烈疼痛,影响口服)
• 支持治疗[b]:轻微症状时基本的口腔护理和症状处理(糖皮质激素漱口水) • 不改变饮食习惯 • 继续使用 mTOR 抑制剂 • 监测病情严重度的变化	• 症状处理和支持治疗[b]:基础口腔护理,局部糖皮质激素,光生物调节(LLLT),改良饮食 • 剂量调整: - 如果毒性可以耐受,无须调整剂量 - 如果毒性无法耐受,①暂时中断给药,直到恢复到≤1 级;②以相同剂量重新启动治疗 - 如果毒性在 2 级复发,①当作第 1 次爆发 3 级管理,中断治疗,直到恢复到≤1 级;②以较低剂量重新开始(即依维莫司 5 mg/d) • 监测病情严重度的变化	• 症状管理和支持治疗[b]:基本口腔护理、系统糖皮质激素、光生物调节、吗啡漱口水、改良饮食、全身镇痛药 • 剂量调整: - 暂时中断给药,直到恢复到≤1 级;以较低剂量重新启动治疗 - 如果毒性在 3 级复发,按照 4 级管理;考虑停药 • 监测病情严重度的变化

来源:Vigarios E,et al. Support Care Cancer,2017,25:1713-1739。获得许可。
a:分级依据 NCI CTCAE V4.0。b:基本口腔护理,见表 8-3。

2. 味觉改变

在接受依维莫司治疗的患者中,多达 1/3 的患者主诉味觉障碍[4],但可能被低估了[23,51],通常不需要调整剂量。由于缺乏标准化的预防和治疗措施,处理(见表 8-3、表 8-4)依靠对症饮食支持。

3. 口腔干燥

在依维莫司治疗的患者中偶有轻度口干的报道(约 6%)[4]。

(二) HER 抑制剂

HER 抑制剂治疗家族包括单克隆抗体(西妥昔单抗、帕尼单抗)和酪氨酸激酶抑制剂(吉非替尼、厄洛替尼)靶向 EGF 受体(表皮生长因子受体,HER1),以及 MKI(阿法替尼、拉帕替尼和达可替尼)抑制 EGFR 和其他 HER(或 ErbB)受体(见表 8-1)[4,35,52-58]。

1. 黏膜炎

(1) 发病率

• EGFR/HER1:在单药治疗中,厄洛替尼和吉非替尼诱发黏膜炎的所有级别发病率分别为 8%～20% 和 19%～24%[4]。此外,高级别(≥3 级)黏膜炎的发病率从未被报道＞1%,不论厄洛替尼还是吉非替尼。

• 泛 HER:相反,在新一代泛 HER 中,黏膜炎似乎是仅次于甲沟炎、腹泻和丘疹脓疱性皮疹的主要毒性之一[52]。阿法替尼引起的全级别黏膜炎的发病率明显高于厄洛替尼或吉非替尼,发病率为29%～64%。达科替尼报道的全级别发病率似乎与阿法替尼非常相似(约40%)。最后,阿法替尼和达科替尼引起的高级别(≥3级)黏膜炎可能在3%～7%的受治患者中发生[4]。

- 针对EGFR的单克隆抗体:与酪氨酸激酶抑制剂相比,西妥昔单抗或帕尼单抗单药治疗的黏膜炎发生率似乎更低[53]。在一项Ⅲ期对照研究中,使用西妥昔单抗治疗患者的全级别黏膜炎发病率为7%,使用帕尼单抗治疗患者的全级别黏膜炎发病率为5%(两组3级黏膜炎发病率均<1%)。
- 西妥昔单抗或帕尼单抗联合化疗:西妥昔单抗和帕尼单抗很少作为单一疗法使用,通常与化疗方案和/或放疗联合使用。与单独化疗相比,西妥昔单抗和帕尼单抗联合化疗均显著增加任何级别黏膜炎的风险[54]。
- 西妥昔单抗与头颈部放疗联合:当西妥昔单抗与放疗联合使用时,高级别(≥3级)黏膜炎的发病率也很高,特别是用于治疗晚期头颈部肿瘤(约60%)[55]。然而,最初主要的关键研究报道,与单独放疗相比,西妥昔单抗加入放疗对高级别(≥3级)黏膜炎的发病率没有显著影响。然而,我们的经验和其他作者的经验[56]表明,这种联合治疗通常观察到更高的重度黏膜炎的发病率。当西妥昔单抗与头颈部放化疗联合使用与不使用西妥昔单抗的头颈部放化疗相比较时,观察到同样的趋势。最后,在头颈部肿瘤中,当西妥昔单抗与放疗联合使用时,高级别(≥3级)黏膜炎的发病率似乎也高于化疗与放疗联合使用[4]。

(2)临床表现 在临床上,黏膜炎相当于中度红斑,有时在治疗开始后不久出现局限的浅表溃疡[4,35,56,57]。它可以表现为阿弗他样病变(图8-6a～c),尽管这些病变比之前描述

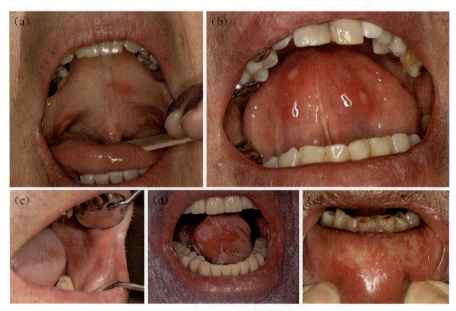

图8-6 HER抑制剂所致黏膜炎

(a)泛HER抑制剂阿法替尼诱导的浅表溃疡,累及非角化黏膜(软腭);(b)黏膜炎,舌腹侧边界清楚的阿弗他样病变(厄洛替尼);(c)单药西妥昔单抗诱导的颊黏膜局限性黏膜炎;(d)3级黏膜炎,西妥昔单抗联合头颈部放疗(见相关的口周放射性皮炎);(e)帕尼单抗联合化疗(卡铂、5-氟尿嘧啶、西妥昔单抗),观察到唇黏膜弥漫性黏膜炎。

的 mTOR 抑制剂所致的病变更不典型。可累及所有非角化区域。值得注意的是，嘴唇病变很常见，包括红斑、糜烂、皲裂[52]和口角炎[58]。

在头颈部放疗中加入西妥昔单抗治疗局部晚期鳞状细胞癌与累及非角化和角化区域的严重病变相关（图 8-6d）。这些病变通常是多发性和多环状的，并常伴明显的功能障碍和口腔周围放射性皮炎。有趣的是，尽管黏膜变化有限，但患者可能会主诉黏膜疼痛。靶向 EGFR 的单克隆抗体与化疗的联合治疗也与较严重的黏膜损伤有关（图 8-6e）。

（3）处理　对于由 HER 抑制剂引起的黏膜炎的预防和治疗处理建议与之前描述的 mIAS 类似（见表 8-3、表 8-4）。有时需要对放疗部分的剂量进行调整，应与相关的肿瘤科医生/放疗科医生密切合作进行讨论。

（4）其他口腔毒性　味觉障碍和口干症多见于新一代 HER 抑制剂（达可替尼、阿法替尼），且大多程度较轻，不需要特别处理[4]。

（三）血管生成抑制剂

血管生成抑制剂类靶向治疗包括直接抑制血管内皮生长因子的单克隆抗体（贝伐珠单抗、雷莫芦单抗）和多激酶抑制剂（舒尼替尼、索拉非尼、帕佐帕尼、阿西替尼、卡博替尼），靶向血管生成受体[VEGF 受体（VEGFR）、血小板衍生生长因子受体（PDGFR）]和其他不同的信号通路（见表 8-1）[4,35,37,38,53,59-65]。

1. 口腔炎

（1）发病率　在接受多靶向血管生成抑制剂治疗的患者中，约 25% 的患者在治疗前 2 个月内发生口腔炎[4,37,59]。在主要的关键性研究中，病变取决于所使用的药物，血管生成抑制剂引起的所有级别的口腔炎发病率为 7%～29%。然而，舒尼替尼、索拉非尼或新注册的卡博替尼更容易引起口腔炎。对照研究表明，全级别血管生成抑制剂相关口腔炎的发病率低于全级别 mIAS[38,60]。

对于舒尼替尼，口腔炎似乎是最常见的不良事件之一（位列腹泻、疲劳和恶心之后），全级别的发生率为 22%～27%[61]。后者似乎高于其他第 1 代多靶点血管生成抑制剂相关的口腔炎，特别是索拉非尼，据报道其所有级别口腔炎的发生率为 7%～19%[4]。使用卡博替尼的所有级别的发生率与使用舒尼替尼的发生率相似，据报道有 22%～29% 的受治患者（60 例）发生口腔炎。

使用任何多靶点血管生成抑制剂，报道高级别（≥3 级）口腔炎的发生率从未超过 4%[60,61]（见表 8-1）。

（2）临床表现　这个广义的术语"口腔炎"被用于描述一系列与血管生成抑制剂相关的黏膜损伤或毒性（如黏膜敏感、味觉改变、口干和口腔溃疡）[12,37]。然而，使用多靶点血管生成抑制剂观察到的口腔改变主要相当于弥漫性黏膜超敏/感觉不良[37]，在一些病例中伴有中度红斑[38]（图 8-7a）或口腔黏膜疼痛性炎症（包括口腔灼烧感，辛辣食物引起的不适）[37]。不太常见的是，非角化黏膜的局限性溃疡（图 8-7b）或可能报道过的线性溃疡，尤其是舒尼替尼或索拉非尼[4,35,59]，治疗开始后（治疗的最初几周）发病迅速，然后逐渐消失[37,38,62]。

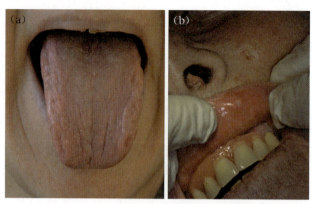

图 8-7 血管生成抑制剂所致口腔炎

(a)卡博替尼治疗患者感觉异常的典型临床表现;(b)用多激酶血管生成抑制剂舒尼替尼观察到局限性口疮样溃疡。

黏膜超敏反应的处理依赖于与 mIAS 或 EGFR 抑制剂诱导的黏膜炎相同的干预措施,以及相关的饮食措施[4](表 8-4)。然而,只有很少患者需要调整剂量(<10%的受治患者)或停止治疗(约 1%的受治患者)[37,59]。

2. 味觉改变

味觉改变似乎是多靶点抗血管生成激酶抑制剂引起的第二常见的口腔不良事件[37]。舒尼替尼和卡博替尼是最常见的两种药物。在这两种药物的治疗中,所有等级的味觉障碍的发生率分别为 20%~49%和 24%~34%(60 例)。高级别味觉障碍显然并不常见,发生在<1%的受治患者中。然而,对照研究表明,与使用 mTOR 抑制剂的患者相比,使用血管生成抑制剂的患者更容易出现味觉障碍[4]。

建议的治疗方案见表 8-3、表 8-4。

3. 良性游走性舌炎

单克隆抗体贝伐珠单抗(图 8-8a)和多激酶血管生成抑制剂[舒尼替尼(图 8-8b)、索拉非尼、阿西替尼等]均可观察到诱发的良性游走性舌炎。通常不需要特殊处理(表 8-7),患者只需安心。在治疗停止后的几个月内,通常会发现病变逐渐消失[63,64]。

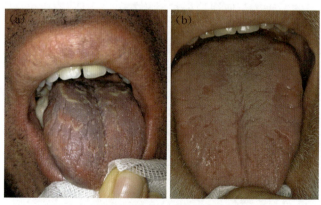

图 8-8 血管生成抑制剂所致良性游走性舌炎

(a)贝伐珠单抗和(b)舒尼替尼诱导的。

4. 其他口腔毒性

根据不同资料,接受多靶点血管生成抑制剂治疗的患者中,有4%～12%的患者会出现1～2级口干症[4]。出血事件和伤口愈合延迟也与这些药物有关,在口腔手术前应全面考虑到这一点。

舒尼替尼和泛RAF抑制剂索拉非尼分别有典型的口腔黏膜黄色变色和局部角化过度病变的报道(图8-9)。

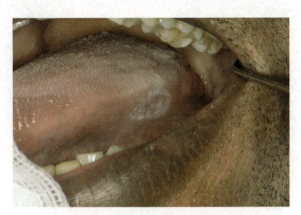

图8-9 多激酶血管生成抑制剂索拉非尼的局部角化过度病变(具有泛RAF抑制活性)

抗再吸收药物[双膦酸盐,如唑来膦酸、帕米膦酸盐、RANKL(NK-κB受体激活剂配体)抑制剂地诺单抗]与抗血管生成靶向治疗(舒尼替尼,贝伐珠单抗)明显增加了药物相关颌骨坏死的风险[65]。最常发生在口腔手术后(见表8-1、表8-7)。

(四) BCR-ABL抑制剂:伊马替尼

1. 口腔苔藓样反应

伊马替尼引发口腔苔藓样反应(图8-10)是该药最常见的个体口腔不良事件(见表8-1)[66-69]。也应进行系统筛查,是否同时累及指甲或皮肤。病变通常为多形性,呈网状条纹,伴有白色丘疹、糜烂或萎缩。主要分布在颊或舌黏膜上。这些病变在经几个月的治疗后逐渐发展,通常是无症状的。因此,需要对伊马替尼治疗的患者进行系统的口腔检查(见表8-7)。一般不需要调整剂量。然而,由于潜在的恶变风险,前瞻性随访是必须的。

2. 色素改变

在接受伊马替尼治疗的患者中,可以发现一种相当典型的"蓝灰色"无症状的硬腭色素沉着(图8-11)[70,71]。口腔其他部位的色素沉着在一些病例报道中也有描述[71]。其病理生理机制与抗疟药物所致色素沉着(药物代谢产物沉积于黏膜,与含铁血黄素或黑色素形成复合物)相似。一些作者认为伊马替尼直接抑制c-KIT(在口腔黏膜中有生理表达)也与这一机制有关。

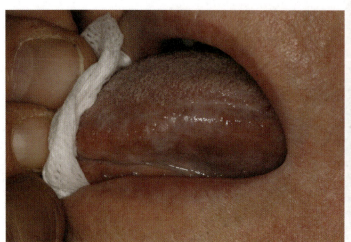
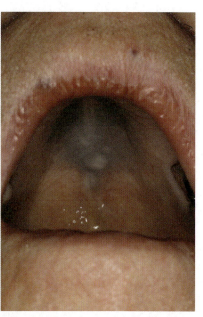

图 8-10　典型苔藓样反应,舌外侧可见网状条纹(伊马替尼)　　图 8-11　伊马替尼引起硬腭相当典型的"蓝灰色"色素沉着

据我们所知,这些口腔变化直到新一代 Bcr-Abl 抑制剂(尼洛替尼、达沙替尼、帕纳替尼)出现前还从未被描述过。

(五) BRAF 抑制剂

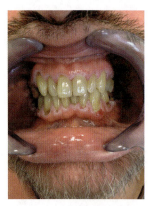

图 8-12　使用 BRAF 抑制剂(维莫非尼)的牙龈缘角化过度病变

在单药治疗中,BRAF 抑制剂(维莫非尼、达拉菲尼、康奈非尼)所引起的皮肤角化过度病变(如疣状乳头状瘤、手足皮肤反应、毛周角化样皮疹、角化棘皮瘤和鳞状细胞癌)是观察到的最常见的皮肤毒性[72](见表 8-1)[72-74]。少见的多灶性无症状的黏膜角化过度病变也已被发现。这些病变主要位于白线、牙龈缘(图 8-12)和硬腭。这些口腔角化过度恶变为鳞状细胞癌虽然罕见,但也是可能的[73](见表 8-7)。因此,对单药治疗的患者应定期进行口腔随访。然而,BRAF 抑制剂目前主要与 MEK 抑制剂(维莫非尼-考比替尼、达拉非尼-曲美替尼)联合使用。通过阻断下游 MAP 激酶通路,MEK 抑制剂明显限制继发性皮肤或黏膜角化过度病变的发展。

最后,使用维莫非尼也曾被报道过有牙龈增生[74]。

(六) 选择性泛 FGFR 抑制剂

口干症是新的选择性泛 FGFR 抑制剂(正在发展中)报道的最常见的治疗诱发的不良事件之一,可能影响 20%~45%的受治患者[75,76]。根据我们的经验,口干症通常为 3 级(图

8-13),可使患者衰弱并严重损害其生活质量[77]。干眼症和皮肤干燥通常相关[76]。此外,选择性 FGFR 抑制剂通常也会引起味觉障碍、粗长的毛发改变和严重的甲剥离[77]。

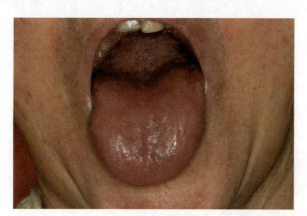

图 8-13　新型选择性泛 FGFR 抑制剂诱导的 3 级口干症

(七) 恩美曲妥珠单抗

抗体偶联药物恩美曲妥珠单抗(TDM-1)使用中已经观察到皮肤和黏膜毛细血管扩张症,与 Osler-Weber-Rendu 综合征相似(见表 8-1)[78,79]。它们表现为蜘蛛状皮肤毛细血管扩张和穹顶状黏膜病变,周围有小的放射状扩张血管(图 8-14)。在这种情况下,建议定期筛查黏膜毛细血管扩张症(见表 8-7)。

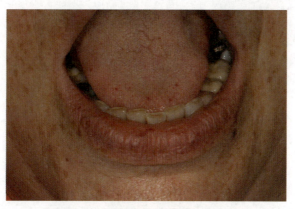

图 8-14　多发黏膜毛细血管扩张累及唇舌(TDM-1)

(八) ALK 抑制剂

10%～25% 克唑替尼治疗的患者可能出现轻至中度的味觉障碍。报道约 15% 的患者出现了全级口炎(无任何 3 级)(见表 8-1)[80]。

(九) Hedgehog 通路抑制剂

在肌痉挛之后,味觉改变是维莫德吉最常见的毒性报道。根据不同的队列,分别有 51%～84% 和 22% 的经治患者分别出现 1～2 级味觉障碍和失聪(见表 8-1)[81,82]。约 5% 的经治患者中断治疗。处理(见表 8-3、表 8-4)依赖于对患者的主动教育,包括营养咨询、保持良好的口腔健康和严格的体重曲线随访。

五 免疫检查点抑制剂

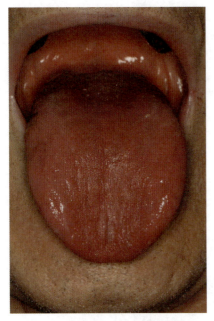

图 8-15 免疫检查点抑制剂所致 3 级口干(纳武单抗)

迄今为止,在临床试验中,免疫检查点抑制剂引起的口腔改变受到的关注有限,尽管最近出现了一系列相关的口腔不良事件[5-7,83-92]。针对 PD-1(尼鲁单抗、派姆单抗)或 PD-L1(阿替利珠单抗、德瓦鲁单抗、阿维单抗)的免疫检查点抑制剂的使用已被发现与偶发病例中的非特异性中度口腔炎或口腔黏膜炎相关[7,85,86]。最近,更多的特征性口腔病变已被描述[5,6,87-92]。

(一) 口干症

据报道,大约 5% 使用抗 PD-1/PD-L1 抗体治疗的患者出现轻至中度口干[83-85]。然而,在一些病例中也可以观察到严重的 3 级口干(图 8-15)。黏膜活检显示 Gougerot-Sjögren 样综合征的组织病理学特征,副唾液腺周围有细胞毒性 T($CD4^+$/$CD8^+$)淋巴细胞浸润(图 8-16)。然而,抗 SSA 和抗 SSB 抗体的检测通常为阴性。

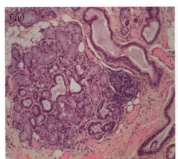 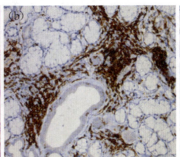 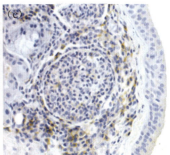

图 8-16 免疫检查点抑制剂所致病变黏膜病理

(a) 唾液腺周围淋巴组织细胞浸润(HE,×10);(b) 免疫染色显示 $CD4^+$ T 细胞浸润(原图放大 20 倍);(c) PD-L1 免疫染色(原图放大 20 倍)。图片由法国 IUCT Colombat 博士提供。

Goujerot-Sjögren 综合征的发生或恶化也偶有与抗 PD-1 有关的报道(同时有关节痛、干燥综合征、抗核抗体和抗 SSA 抗体阳性)[5]。

处理依据表 8-3 和表 8-4 所述的支持措施。

(二) 味觉障碍

有不到 3% 的采用抗 PD-1 和 PD-L1 药物的患者出现中度味觉障碍。口干症和味觉障碍在抗 CTLA-4 药物伊匹单抗中较少见。

(三) 口腔苔藓样反应

鉴于其作为触发 T 细胞激活的免疫调节剂的作用机制,免疫检查点抑制剂与特定的毒性相关,主要是基于免疫机制的性质[5,92]。因此,在引入抗-PD1/PD-L1 治疗几个月后观察到口腔苔藓样反应并不罕见[5,90-92],这强烈表明存在类效应[92]。病变通常以孤立的方式发生,但皮肤、指甲或肛周/生殖器区域也可同时受损伤[5,91,92]。

口腔检查显示在舌头(图 8-17a)、颊黏膜(图 8-17b)、上颚(图 8-17c)和唇内侧/牙龈黏膜[92]上呈对称网状白色条纹,与 Wickham 纹一致。也可观察到丘疹、斑块样、溃疡性或萎缩性/红斑性病变,有时合并出现,可影响角化和非角化黏膜。这些诱发的苔藓样病变通常是自限性和低级别的。组织学上,真皮表皮交界处可见中度带状淋巴组织细胞浸润,伴斑片状至花簇状空泡化界面性皮炎;基底膜区部分破裂;细胞凋亡、颗粒增生和角化不全[92]。

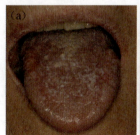 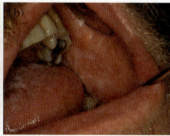 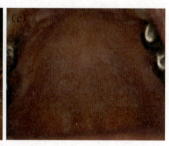

图 8-17 免疫检查点抑制剂所致口腔苔藓样病变

(a)涉及舌头背侧的口腔苔藓样反应(尼鲁单抗);(b)颊黏膜和舌背的点状和网状苔藓样病变(尼鲁单抗);(c)腭部出现广泛的网状苔藓样病变(尼鲁单抗)。

口腔苔藓样病变没有报道导致停止或中断肿瘤治疗,并且,在大多数情况下,它们在外用糖皮质激素(氯倍他索软膏或乳膏、地塞米松/泼尼龙漱口水)治疗数周后症状改善。通常观察到停止治疗后病变完全消失[92]。对于苔藓样病变恶化的潜在风险,需要定期随访[88,92],对于不典型病变推荐活检(见表 8-3、表 8-4)。

(四) 其他毒性

抗 PD1 或抗 PD-L1 药物已被证明会导致免疫相关大疱性类天疱疮的风险升高,有时会累及口腔黏膜[5]。

参 考 文 献

1. Lalla RV, Saunders DP, Peterson DE. Chemotherapy or radiation-induced oral mucositis. *Dent Clin North Am* 2014;58:341-9.
2. Staudenmaier T et al. Burden of oral mucositis in stem cell transplant patients-the patients' perspective. *Support Care Cancer* Epub December 2,2017.
3. Barkokebas A et al. Impact of oral mucositis on oral health-related quality of life of patients diagnosed with cancer. *J Oral Pathol Med* 2015;44:746-51.
4. Vigarios E, Epstein JB, Sibaud V. Oral mucosal changes induced by anticancer targeted therapies and immune checkpoint inhibitors. *Support Care Cancer* 2017;25:1713-39.
5. Sibaud V. Dermatologic reactions to immune checkpoint inhibitors: Skin toxicities and immunotherapy. *Am J Clin Dermatol* 2018;19:345-61.
6. Jackson LK et al. Oral health in oncology: Impact of immunotherapy. *Support Care Cancer* 2015;23:1-3.
7. Freeman-Keller M et al. Nivolumab in resected and unresecable metastatic melanoma: Characteristics of immune-related adverse events and association with outcomes. *Clin Cancer Res* 2016;22:886-94.
8. Peterson DE, Srivastava R, Lalla RV. Oral mucosal injury in oncology patients: Perspectives on maturation of a field. *Oral Dis* 2015;21:133-41.
9. Cinausero M et al. New frontiers in the pathobiology and treatment of cancer regimen-related mucosal injury. *Front Pharmacol* 2017;8:354.
10. Sonis ST. The pathobiology of mucositis. *Nat Rev Cancer* 2004;4:277-84.
11. Moslemi D et al. Management of chemo/radiation-induced oral mucositis in patients with head and neck cancer: A review of the current literature. *Radiother Oncol* 2016;120:13-20.
12. Al-Ansari S et al. Oral mucositis induced by anticancer therapies. *Curr Oral Health Rep* 2015;2:202-11.
13. Chaveli-López B. Oral toxicity produced by chemotherapy: A systematic review. *J Clin Exp Dent* 2014;6: e81-90.
14. Elad S, Zadik Y, Yarom N. Oral complications of nonsurgical cancer therapies. *Atlas Oral Maxillofac Surg Clin North Am* 2017;25:133-47.
15. Raber-Durlacher JE, Elad S, Barasch A. Oral mucositis. *Oral Oncol* 2010;46:452-6.
16. Peterson DE et al. Management of oral and gastrointestinal mucosal injury: ESMO Clinical Practice Guidelines for diagnosis, treatment, and follow-up. *Ann Oncol* 2015;26 Suppl 5: v139-51.
17. Lalla RV et al. Mucositis guidelines leadership group of the multinational association of supportive care in cancer and international society of oral oncology (MASCC/ISOO). MASCC/ISOO clinical practice guidelines for the management of mucositis secondary to cancer therapy. *Cancer* 2014;120:1453-61.
18. De Sanctis V et al. Mucositis in head and neck cancer patients treated with radiotherapy and systemic therapies: Literature review and consensus statements. *Crit Rev Oncol Hematol* 2016;100:147-66.
19. Elad S et al. Basic oral care for hematology-oncology patients and hematopoietic stem cell transplantation recipients: A position paper from the joint task force of the Multinational Association of Supportive Care in Cancer/International Society of Oral Oncology (MASCC/ISOO) and the European Society for Blood and Marrow Transplantation (EBMT). *Support Care Cancer* 2015;23:223-36.

20. Zecha JA et al. Low-level laser therapy/photobiomodulation in the management of side effects of chemoradiation therapy in head and neck cancer: Part 2: Proposed applications and treatment protocols. *Support Care Cancer* 2016;24:2793-805.
21. Bronner AK, Hood AF. Cutaneous complications of chemotherapeutic agents. *J Am Acad Dermatol* 1983;9:645-63.
22. Sibaud V et al. Pigmentary disorders induced by anticancer agents. Part I: Chemotherapy. *Ann Dermatol Venereol* 2013;140:183-96.
23. Epstein JB, Smutzer G, Doty RL. Understanding the impact of taste changes in oncology care. *Support Care Cancer* 2016;24:1917-31.
24. Ponticelli E et al. Dysgeusia and health-related quality of life of cancer patients receiving chemotherapy: A cross-sectional study. *Eur J Cancer Care* 2017;26(2).
25. Sibaud V et al. Dermatological adverse events with taxane chemotherapy. *Eur J Dermatol* 2016;26:427-43.
26. Van der Veen J, Nuyts S. Can intensity-modulated-radiotherapy reduce toxicity in head and neck squamous cell carcinoma? *Cancer* 2017;9(10).
27. Sroussi HY et al. Common oral complications of head and neck cancer radiation therapy: Mucositis, infections, saliva change, fibrosis, sensory dysfunctions, dental caries, periodontal disease, and osteoradionecrosis. *Cancer Med* Epub October 25.2017.
28. Maria OM, Eliopoulos N, Muanza T. Radiation-induced oral mucositis. *Front Oncol* 2017;7:89.
29. Elad S, Zadik Y. Chronic oral mucositis after radiotherapy to the head and neck: A new insight. *Support Care Cancer* 2016;24:4825-30.
30. Hartl DM et al. Otorhinolaryngological toxicities of new drugs in oncology. *Adv Ther* 2017;34:866-94.
31. de Bataille C et al. Management of radiation-induced mucosal necrosis with photobiomodulation therapy. *Support Care Cancer* Epub October 9,2017.
32. Mercadante V et al. Interventions for the management of radiotherapy-induced xerostomia and hyposalivation: A systematic review and meta-analysis. *Oral Oncol* 2017;66:64-74.
33. Buglione M et al. Oral toxicity management in head and neck cancer patients treated with chemotherapy and radiation: Xerostomia and trismus (Part 2). Literature review and consensus statement. *Crit Rev Oncol Hematol* 2016;102:47-54.
34. Yang WF et al. Is pilocarpine effective in preventing radiation-induced xerostomia? A systematic review and meta-analysis. *Int J Radiat Oncol Biol Phys* 2016;94:503-11.
35. Sibaud V et al. Oral toxicity of targeted anticancer therapies. *Ann Dermatol Venereol* 2014;141:354-63.
36. Watters AL, Epstein JB, Agulnik M. Oral complications of targeted cancer therapies: A narrative literature review. *Oral Oncol* 2011;47:441-8.
37. Yuan A et al. Oral adverse events in cancer patients treated with VEGFR-directed multitargeted tyrosine kinase inhibitors. *Oral Oncol* 2015;51:1026-33.
38. Boers-Doets CB et al. Oral adverse events associated with tyrosine kinase and mammalian target of rapamycin inhibitors in renal cell carcinoma: A structured literature review. *Oncologist* 2012;17:135-44.
39. Peterson DE et al. Oral mucosal injury caused by mammalian target of rapamycin inhibitors: Emerging perspectives on pathobiology and impact on clinical practice. *Cancer Med* 2016;5:1897-907.
40. Jensen SB, Peterson DE. Oral mucosal injury caused by cancer therapies: Current management and new frontiers in research. *J Oral Pathol Med* 2014;43:81-90.

41. Yuan A, Woo SB. Adverse drug events in the oral cavity. *Oral Surg Oral Med Oral Path Oral Rad* 2015;119:35-47.
42. Reyes-Habito CM, Roh EK. Cutaneous reactions to chemotherapeutic drugs and targeted therapy for cancer: Part II. Targeted therapy. *J Am Acad Dermatol* 2014;71:217. e1-217. e11.
43. Sonis S et al. Preliminary characterization of oral lesions associated with inhibitors of mammalian target of rapamycin in cancer patients. *Cancer* 2010;116:210-5.
44. Martins F et al. A review of oral toxicity associated with mTOR inhibitor therapy in cancer patients. *Oral Oncol* 2013;49:293-8.
45. Gomez-Fernandez C et al. The risk of skin rash and stomatitis with the mammalian target of rapamycin inhibitor temsirolimus: A systematic review of the literature and meta-analysis. *Eur J Cancer* 2012;48:340-6.
46. Vargo CA et al. Occurrence and characterization of everolimus adverse events during first and subsequent cycles in the treatment of metastatic breast cancer. *Support Care Cancer* 2016;24:2913-8.
47. Rugo HS et al. Incidence and time course of everolimus-related adverse events in postmenopausal women with hormone receptor-positive advanced breast cancer: Insights from BOLERO-2. *Ann Oncol* 2014;25:808-15.
48. De Oliveira MA et al. Clinical presentation and management of mTOR inhibitor-associated stomatitis. *Oral Oncol* 2011;47:998-1003.
49. Rugo HS et al. Meta-analysis of stomatitis in clinical studies of everolimus: Incidence and relationship with efficacy. *Ann Oncol* 2016;27:519-25.
50. Rugo HS et al. Prevention of everolimus-related stomatitis in women with hormone receptor-positive, HER2-negative metastatic breast cancer using dexamethasone mouthwash (SWISH): A single-arm, phase 2 trial. *Lancet Oncol* 2017;18:654-62.
51. Macdonald JB, Macdonald B, Golitz LE, LoRusso P, Sekulic A. Cutaneous adverse effects of targeted therapies: Part II: Inhibitors of intracellular molecular signaling pathways. *J Am Acad Dermatol* 2015;72(2):221-36.
52. Melosky B, Hirsh V. Management of common toxicities in metastatic NSCLC related to anti-lung cancer therapies with EGFR-TKIs. *Front Oncol* 2014;4:238.
53. Elting LS et al. Risk of oral and gastrointestinal mucosal injury among patients receiving selected targeted agents: A meta-analysis. *Support Care Cancer* 2013;21:3243-54.
54. Miroddi M et al. Risk of grade 3-4 diarrhea and mucositis in colorectal cancer patients receiving anti-EGFR monoclonal antibodies regimens: A meta-analysis of 18 randomized controlled clinical trials. *Crit Rev Oncol Hematol* 2015;96:355-71.
55. Bonner JA et al. Radiotherapy plus cetuximab for squamous-cell carcinoma of the head and neck. *N Engl J Med* 2006;354:567-78.
56. Tejwani A et al. Increased risk of high-grade dermatologic toxicities with radiation plus epidermal growth factor receptor inhibitor therapy. *Cancer* 2009;115:1286-99.
57. Lacouture ME et al. Clinical practice guidelines for the prevention and treatment of EGFR inhibitor-associated dermatologic toxicities. *Support Care Cancer* 2011;19:1079-95.
58. Lacouture ME et al. A proposed EGFR inhibitor dermatologic adverse event-specific grading scale from the MASCC skin toxicity study group. *Support Care Cancer* 2010;18:509-22.
59. Kollmannsberger C et al. Sunitinib in metastatic renal cell carcinoma: Recommendations for management of non-cardiovascular toxicities. *Oncologist* 2011;16:543-53.
60. Elisei R et al. Cabozantinib in progressive medullary thyroid cancer. *J Clin Oncol* 2013;31:3639-46.
61. Ibrahim EM et al. Sunitinib adverse events in metastatic renal cell carcinoma: A meta-analysis. *Int J*

Clin Oncol 2013;18:1060-9.
62. Edmonds K et al. Strategies for assessing and managing the adverse events of sorafenib and other targeted therapies in the treatment of renal cell and hepatocellular carcinoma: Recommendations from a European nursing task group. *Eur J Oncol Nurs* 2012;16:172-84.
63. Gavrilovic IT et al. Characteristics of oral mucosal events related to bevacizumab treatment. *Oncologist* 2012;17:274-8.
64. Hubiche T et al. Geographic tongue induced by angiogenesis inhibitors. *Oncologist* 2013;18: e16-17.
65. Christodoulou C et al. Combination of bisphosphonates and antiangiogenic factors induces osteonecrosis of the jaw more frequently than bisphosphonates alone. *Oncology* 2009;76:209-11.
66. Gómez Fernández C et al. Oral lichenoid eruption associated with imatinib treatment. *Eur J Dermatol* 2010;20:127-8.
67. Amitay-Laish I, Stemmer SM, Lacouture ME. Adverse cutaneous reactions secondary to tyrosine kinase inhibitors including imatinib mesylate, nilotinib, and dasatinib. *Dermatol Ther* 2011;24: 386-95.
68. Basso FG et al. Skin and oral lesions associated to imatinib mesylate therapy. *Support Care Cancer* 2009;17:465-8.
69. Fitzpatrick SG, Hirsch SA, Gordon SC. The malignant transformation of oral lichen planus and oral lichenoid lesions: A systematic review. *J Am Dent Assoc* 2014;145:45-56.
70. Khoo TL et al. Hyperpigmentation of the hard palate associated with imatinib therapy for chronic myeloid leukemia with a genetic variation in the proto-oncogene c-KIT. *Leuk Lymphoma* 2013;54: 186-8.
71. Balagula Y et al. Pigmentary changes in a patient treated with imatinib. *J Drugs Dermatol* 2011;10: 1062-6.
72. Boussemart L et al. Prospective study of cutaneous side-effects associated with the BRAF inhibitor vemurafenib: A study of 42 patients. *Ann Oncol* 2013;24:1691-7.
73. Vigarios E et al. Oral squamous cell carcinoma and hyperkeratotic lesions with BRAF inhibitors. *Br J Dermatol* 2015;172:1680-2.
74. Mangold AR, Bryce A, Sekulic A. Vemurafenib-associated gingival hyperplasia in patient with metastatic melanoma. *J Am Acad Dermatol* 2014;71: e205-6.
75. Nogova L et al. Evaluation of BGJ398, a fibroblast growth factor receptor 1-3 kinase inhibitor, in patients with advanced solid tumors harboring genetic alterations in fibroblast growth factor receptors: Results of a global phase I, dose-escalation and dose-expansion study. *J Clin Oncol* 2017;35:157-65.
76. Tabernero J et al. Phase I dose-escalation study of JNJ-42756493, an oral pan-fibroblast growth factor receptor inhibitor, in patients with advanced solid tumors. *J Clin Oncol* 2015;33:3401-8.
77. Bétrian S et al. Severe onycholysis and eyelash trichomegaly following use of new selective pan-FGFR inhibitors. *JAMA Dermatol* 2017;153:723-5.
78. Sibaud V et al. Ado-trastuzumab emtansine-associated telangiectasias in metastatic breast cancer: A case series. *Breast Cancer Res Treat* 2014;146:423-6.
79. Sibaud V et al. T-DM1-related telangiectasias: A potential role in secondary bleeding events. *Ann Oncol* 2015;26:436-7.
80. Solomon BJ et al. First-line crizotinib versus chemotherapy in ALK-positive lung cancer. *N Engl J Med* 2014;371:2167-77.
81. Basset-Seguin N et al. Vismodegib in patients with advanced basal cell carcinoma (STEVIE): A pre-planned interim analysis of an international, open-label trial. *Lancet Oncol* 2015;16:729-36.
82. Sekulic A et al. Efficacy and safety of vismodegib in advanced basal-cell carcinoma. *N Engl J Med*

2012;366:2171-9.
83. Rizvi NA et al. Activity and safety of nivolumab, an anti-PD-1 immune checkpoint inhibitor, for patients with advanced, refractory squamous non-small-cell lung cancer (CheckMate 063): A phase 2, single-arm trial. *Lancet Oncol* 2015;16:257-65.
84. Topalian SL et al. Survival, durable tumor remission, and long-term safety in patients with advanced melanoma receiving nivolumab. *J Clin Oncol* 2014;32:1020-30.
85. McDermott DF et al. Atezolizumab, an anti-programmed death-ligand 1 antibody, in metastatic renal cell carcinoma: Long-term safety, clinical activity, and immune correlates from a phase Ia study. *J Clin Oncol* 2016;34:833-42.
86. Haanen JBAG et al. Management of toxicities from immunotherapy: ESMO Clinical Practice Guidelines for diagnosis, treatment and follow-up. *Ann Oncol* 2017;28: iv119-42.
87. Shi VJ et al. Clinical and histologic features of lichenoid mucocutaneous eruptions due to anti-programmed cell death 1 and anti-programmed cell death ligand 1 immunotherapy. *JAMA Dermatol* 2016;152:1128-36.
88. Rapoport BL et al. Supportive care for patients undergoing immunotherapy. *Support Care Cancer* Epub July 13,2017.
89. Naidoo J et al. Toxicities of the anti-PD-1 and anti-PD-L1 immune checkpoint antibodies. *Ann Oncol* 2015;26:2375-91.
90. Hofmann L et al. Cutaneous, gastrointestinal, hepatic, endocrine, and renal side-effects of anti-PD-1 therapy. *Eur J Cancer* 2016;60:190-209.
91. Schaberg KB et al. Immunohistochemical analysis of lichenoid reactions in patients treated with anti-PD-L1 and anti-PD-1 therapy. *J Cutan Pathol* 2016;43:339-46.
92. Sibaud V et al. Oral lichenoid reactions associated with anti-PD-1/PD-L1 therapies: Clinicopathological findings. *J Eur Acad Dermatol Venereol* 2017;31: e464-9.

第九章

化疗引起的甲反应

埃里克·王（Eric Wong），玛丽亚·卡梅拉·阿农齐亚塔（Maria Carmela Annunziata），
安东内拉·托斯蒂（Antonella Tosti）

张 颖 译

化疗是甲不良反应的常见病因。甲异常通常由急性损伤引起，其临床特点取决于甲器官的哪个部分受累[1]。甲器官由甲母质、甲床、甲板、甲下皮、近端和外侧甲皱襞组成[2]。甲改变可在暴露于药物后立即发生，也可以在治疗数月后出现。恢复可能很慢，因为指甲和趾甲的甲单位生长速度分别为每月 3 mm 和 1 mm[3]。化疗引起的大多数甲异常累及多个或者所有甲[4]。

症状不一，从无症状到疼痛和不适。在某些情况下，患者因甲改变需要中断治疗[4]。然而，虽然有些改变可能为永久性的，但绝大多数甲异常在停药后可逆转[1]。

一 药物引起的甲母质损伤

引起甲母质角质形成细胞有丝分裂活性急剧减少或停止的药物可导致各种体征，从甲轻度变薄或生长缓慢至甲板完全停止生长[3]，医生应询问在甲出现症状前的 2～3 周开始可能使用的药物。甲改变包括甲变薄/变脆、甲生长速度改变以及甲板停止生长，角质形成细胞有丝分裂活性受损。

（一）甲变薄/变脆

紫杉烷、布鲁顿酪氨酸激酶（Bruton tyrosine kinase, BTK）抑制剂（包括依鲁替尼）和 BRAF 抑制剂（维罗非尼），以及表皮生长因子受体（EGFR）抑制剂等化疗药物可改变甲板的生成，导致甲变薄、变脆（图 9-1）[1,4-7]。虽然化疗引起脆甲的发病机制不明，但有人提出原因是多方面的，包括甲母质破坏导致甲板合成改变、破坏已角化的甲板，或者晚期肿瘤患者可能存在代谢不良或营养不良[1,3,8]。

薄甲及脆甲的治疗包括：戴橡胶手套以避免外伤及反复接触水；保持短甲以维护好日常甲卫

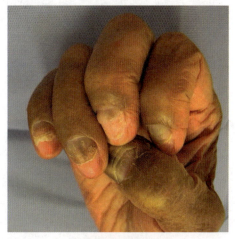

图 9-1 接受厄洛替尼治疗的患者甲脱落、甲分离和脆甲

生;避免刺激物及洗甲水(可导致脱水);使用甲保湿剂(包括封包剂和保湿剂)[9]。口服补充生物素(每日 5 mg),随时间推移,可使甲逐渐强化[10]。美国 FDA 已批准甲油(羟丙基壳聚糖和 16%聚脲氨基甲酸酯)用于治疗脆甲[8]。

(二) 甲生长速度改变

化疗药物,包括甲氨蝶呤,可降低甲生长速度[11],一旦停药,甲生长速度通常会恢复正常[3]。

(三) 博氏线/脱甲症

博氏线表现为发生在甲板上的横向凹陷或压痕(图 9-2)[3,12]。脱甲症,是用于描述较严重博氏线的术语,表现为甲从近端甲皱襞分离或脱落(图 9-1)[19],凹陷的长度和大小可提示医生致病源对甲母质损伤的持续时间及严重程度[1]。通常影响大多数或所有的甲,常表现为多条线,每条线对应一个化疗周期。

最常与甲母质受损有关的化疗药物包括紫杉烷、顺铂、美法仑及长春新碱[1,13-17]。博氏线或脱甲症随着甲的生长而消失[20]。

在患者等待甲长出来期间,治疗通常仅限于缓解症状[11]。

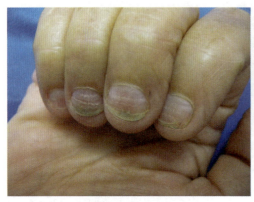

图 9-2　博氏线

表现为甲板横向凹陷,对应每个化疗周期。

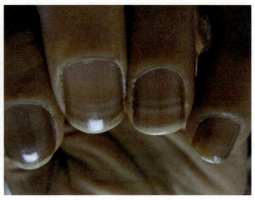

图 9-3　真性白甲

每个化疗周期后出现的横向平行白线。

(四) 真性横向白甲

药物损伤远端甲母质角质形成细胞的有丝分裂活性,导致腹侧甲板角化不全(或细胞核滞留)伴横向白甲。与显性白甲相反(见后文),真性横向白甲表现为不透明、持久的白色条带,通常宽 1~2 mm,随着甲生长而向远端移动(图 9-3),对其施加压力后,条带并不消失[12]。与博氏线相似,甲通常呈多个条带,对应重复的化疗周期。

与真性横向白甲有关的化疗药物包括柔红霉素、多柔比星、环磷酰胺、长春新碱以及治疗急性髓性白血病的砷剂[11]。横向白甲无特殊治疗,甲板随着时间推移会生长出来[3]。

(五) 药物引起的甲色素沉着(黑甲)

黑甲是因甲母质活跃的黑色素细胞产生黑色素,甲板出现纵向或横向分布的黑色或棕色色素沉着(图9-4)[1,3,18,19]。药物引起的黑甲一般累及多个或所有的甲,开始用药后3~8周即出现(图9-5);它可与其他皮肤与黏膜的色素沉着相关,并伴化疗引起的其他甲异常[8]。一旦停止药物治疗,这类颜色改变可以逆转,但需要数周至数月等待甲长出[11]。最常报道引起黑甲的化疗药物包括羟基脲、甲氨蝶呤、博来霉素、环磷酰胺、蒽环类药物(柔红霉素)及5-氟尿嘧啶[8,21]。

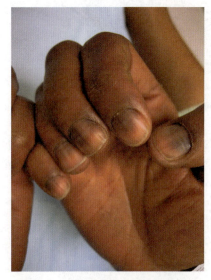 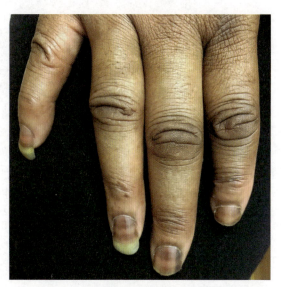

图9-4 1例接受综合化疗患者的马尔克线(Muehrcke line)(显性白甲)及黑甲

图9-5 多柔比星引起的纵向及横向黑甲

由 Beth McLellan 博士提供。

二 药物引起的甲床损伤

(一) 甲分离

甲床受损导致甲板分开形成甲分离(图9-1)。化疗药物引起的甲分离常伴有出血及疼痛[1]。接受紫杉烷治疗的患者中,疼痛性出血性甲分离可继发细菌感染,形成甲下脓肿(图9-6)[20]。这被认为是因为药物对甲床的毒性作用,破坏了血管生成。疼痛是由于压力引起的,人工/手术引流可缓解。甲下脓肿可导致严重的并发症,包括脓毒血症,尤其是在粒细胞缺乏的患者中。由于紫杉烷的免疫抑制作用,其化疗方案被认为增加了细菌感染的易感性[13,22-26]。BRAF抑制剂(达拉菲尼)、卡培他滨、依托泊苷、氟尿嘧啶、米托蒽醌及多柔比星亦可引起甲分离[1,5,8,16,27-30]。

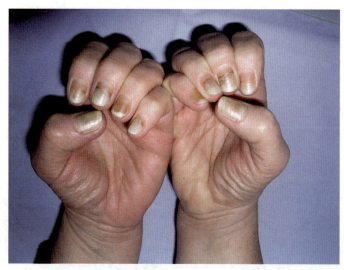

图9-6　1例使用紫杉烷患者的出血性甲分离

一旦停止刺激因素,甲分离通常被认为是可逆的。有时,甲分离可以在不停药的情况下消退。因此,一般对症治疗即可。治疗建议包括:将手指浸泡在抗菌溶液中,以预防继发微生物定植并降低感染率;尽可能剪短没有附着的甲,保持常规的手卫生;洗手后轻柔擦干;避免接触刺激物;戴手套预防和保护,防止外伤[9,11]。

甲下脓肿的治疗,包括使用抗生素和/或环氧合酶-2抑制剂[31]。采用冰的手套或袜子进行低温治疗(温度-30℃),可预防/减少不良反应,避免停用治疗肿瘤的药物[4,32]。

(二) 显性白甲

显性白甲表现为平行分布的白色条带,受压后消失。与真性白甲不同的是,显性白甲不随甲板的生长而迁移[1]。白甲确切的发病机制尚不清楚,但被认为是由甲床血管损伤引起的,导致可变化的血液流量[1,18,11]。马尔克线甲是化疗引起的显性白甲的经典案例(图9-4)[8]。显性白甲是联合化疗常见的不良反应。显性白甲亦见于接受多柔比星和酪氨酸激酶抑制剂(TKI),如索拉非尼、舒尼替尼及伊马替尼治疗的患者[8,33]。显性白甲常在停药后消退[18]。

三　药物引起的近端甲皱襞损伤

(一) 急性甲沟炎

甲沟炎表现为近端或外侧甲皱襞的触痛以及疼痛性炎症[18]。虽然对甲沟炎的发病机制知之甚少,但药物引起的甲沟炎被认为与易碎的甲碎片进入甲周区域有关,通常发生在开始用药后1~3个月内[11]。可引起这种不良反应的化疗药物包括:甲氨蝶呤、MEK抑制剂(包括司美替尼、曲美替尼、考比替尼)、EGFR抑制剂(如帕尼单抗、吉非替尼、西妥昔单抗及拉帕替尼)和治疗转移性黑色素瘤的 BRAF 抑制剂(维罗非尼)[5,34-39]。10%～15%使用这些化疗药物的患者,可发生药物引起的甲沟炎,通常是在治疗开始后 1 个月内[41]。甲沟炎常并发化脓性肉芽肿。

药物减量或停用后,甲沟炎倾向消退;然而,治疗有助于减少炎症,包括适当的甲卫生和保护、抗菌洗液以及局部外用类固醇激素[1,40]。其他治疗包括外用聚维酮碘/二甲基亚砜溶液、化学烧灼(使用硝酸银或亚硫酸铁)、四环素类抗生素、外用阿达帕林、破坏性方法(电蚀)或手术切除(切除部分甲板)[37,38,42-45]。

(二) 化脓性肉芽肿

化脓性肉芽肿表现为小的、圆形、红色有光泽的结节,伴有出血倾向[1],化脓性肉芽肿见于使用紫杉烷、酪氨酸激酶抑制剂(图 9-7)、MEK 抑制剂和 EGFR 抑制剂如西妥昔单抗的患者,通常累及单个或多个甲的近端及外侧甲皱襞[4,8,33,34,37,39]。通常停药后可以改善症状,但有时外用类固醇激素和/或莫匹罗星软膏有助于改善症状及预防感染[11,12],其他可以考虑的治疗包括外用阿利维 A 酸(9-顺式维 A 酸)、8%苯酚溶液烧灼肉芽肿、局部液氮治疗、外用激素或每周 1 次 10%硝酸银水溶液。可行外科切除,但皮损可能复发[8,11,46-48]。根据笔者经验,光动力治疗亦为一种有效的治疗方法。

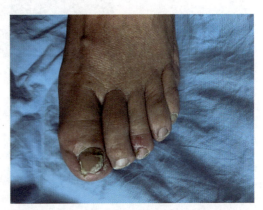

图 9-7　阿法替尼引起的甲沟炎和化脓性肉芽肿

由 Beth McLellan 博士提供。

四　药物引起的甲血流改变

(一) 缺血

组织灌注受损时,会发生缺血,并可能导致坏死。如果血液循环不能恢复,缺血可以从雷诺现象进展为坏疽。雷诺现象是缺血的最初征兆,是动脉血管痉挛导致血流量减少的结果。症状可能是不可逆的,如缺血持续太久,可能需要截肢或截指/趾。系统性或病变内使用博来霉素治疗生殖细胞睾丸癌,可引起末梢肢端和甲的缺血[11,49]。

(二) 甲下出血

甲下出血表现为甲单位的裂片状出血及甲下血肿,是由于甲床血流改变引起甲单位损伤所导致。与血小板减少症相同,裂片状出血被认为是选择性 VEGF 阻滞剂引起甲床内垂直走向的血管形成微小血凝块所致,表现为短小的紫色至棕色线条(图 9-8)[1,19]。裂片状出血通常没有症状,发生在 30%～70%患者中,在开始接受抗 VEGF/VEGFR 药物治疗后

2～4周出现。这些症状可能提示药物治疗有效[53]。甲下血肿是因于甲板与甲床之间红色至棕色出血。这两种病变往往随时间推移而消退[11]。使用紫杉烷、米托蒽醌和包括索拉非尼、舒尼替尼及伊马替尼在内的抗VEGFR药物可出现甲下出血及甲下血肿[26,33,45,51]。

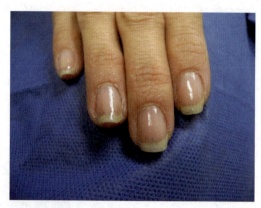

图9-8　1例接受VEGF抑制剂的患者出现甲床裂片状出血

按药物类别总结最常见对甲的不良反应见表9-1。

表9-1　药物种类和最常见的不良反应（按最常见至不常见排序）

药物种类	甲异常	参考文献
EGFR抑制剂	甲沟炎伴化脓性肉芽肿 脆甲	8，36，38，47，52 45
VEFGR抑制剂	裂片状出血 马克尔线	8，33，45 33
TKI类药物	甲沟炎 甲下裂片状出血	36 45
MEK抑制剂	甲沟炎 甲分离	37 5
BRAF抑制剂	甲沟炎 甲分离 脆甲	5
紫杉烷类药物	出血性甲分离伴甲下脓肿 脱甲症/博氏线 甲沟炎 脆甲症	4，13，23，26 50

参 考 文 献

1. Piraccini BM et al. Drug-induced nail diseases. *Dermatol Clin* 2006；24(3)：387－91.
2. Haneke E. Surgical anatomy of the nail apparatus. *Dermatol Clin* 2006；24：291－6.

3. Piraccini BM, Tosti A. Drug-induced nail disorders: Incidence, management and prognosis. *Drug Saf* 1999;21(3):187-201.
4. Gilbar P, Hain A, Peereboom VM. Nail toxicity induced by cancer chemotherapy. *J Oncol Pharm Pract* 2009;15(3):143-55.
5. Dika E et al. Hair and nail adverse events during treatment with targeted therapies for metastatic melanoma. *Eur J Dermatol* 2016;26(3):232-9.
6. Bitar C et al. Hair and nail changes during long-term therapy with ibrutinib for chronic lymphocytic leukemia. *JAMA Dermatol* 2016;152(6):698-701.
7. Garden BC, Wu S, Lacouture ME. The risk of nail changes with epidermal growth factor receptor inhibitors: A systematic review of the literature and meta-analysis. *J Am Acad Dermatol* 2012;67(3): 400-8.
8. Robert C et al. Nail toxicities induced by systemic anticancer treatments. *Lancet Oncol* 2015;16(4): e181-9.
9. Piraccini BM et al. Treatment of nail disorders. *Therapy* 2004;1(1):159-67.
10. Colombo VE et al. Treatment of brittle fingernails and onychoschizia with biotin: Scanning electron microscopy. *J Am Acad Dermatol* 1990;23(6 Pt 1):1127-32.
11. Piraccini BM, Iorizzo M. Drug reactions affecting the nail unit: Diagnosis and management. *Dermatol Clin* 2007;25(2):215-21, vii.
12. Piraccini BM et al. Drug-induced nail abnormalities. *Expert Opin Drug Saf* 2004;3(1):57-65.
13. Minisini AM et al. Taxane-induced nail changes: Incidence, clinical presentation and outcome. *Ann Oncol* 2003;14(2):333-7.
14. Eastwood JB et al. Shedding of nails apparently induced by the administration of large amounts of cephaloridine and cloxacillin in two anephric patients. *Br J Dermatol* 1969;81(10):750-2.
15. Chen HH, Liao YH. Beau's lines associated with itraconazole. *Acta Dermato-Venereologica* 2002;82 (5):398.
16. Susser WS, Whitaker-Worth DL, Grant-Kels JM. Mucocutaneous reactions to chemotherapy. *J Am Acad Dermatol* 1999;40:367-98.
17. Vassallo C et al. Nail changes secondary to hematologic conditions. *Haematologica* 2001;86:334-6.
18. Hinds G, Thomas VD. Malignancy and cancer treatment-related hair and nail changes. *Dermatol Clin* 2008;26(1):59-68, viii.
19. Piraccini BM, Iorizzo M, Tosti A. Drug-induced nail abnormalities. *Am J Clin Dermatol* 2003;4:31-7.
20. Roh MR, Cho JY, Lew W. Docetaxel-induced onycholysis: The role of subungual hemorrhage and suppuration. *Yonsei Med J* 2007;48(1):124-6.
21. Oh ST et al. Hydroxyurea-induced melanonychia concomitant with a dermatomyositis-like eruption. *J Am Acad Dermatol* 2003;49(2):339-41.
22. Vanhooteghem O et al. Subungual abscess: A new ungula side-effect related to docetaxel therapy. *Br J Dermatol* 2000;143(2):462-4.
23. Pavithran K, Doval DC. Nail changes due to docetaxel. *Br J Dermatol* 2002;146(4):709-10.
24. Nicolopoulos J, Howard A. Docetaxel-induced nail dystrophy. *Australas J Dermatol* 2002;43(3): 293-6.
25. Correia O et al. Nail changes secondary to docetaxel (Taxotere). *Dermatology* 1999;198(3):288-90.
26. Ghetti E, Piraccini BM, Tosti A. Onycholysis and subungual haemorrhages secondary to systemic chemotherapy (paclitaxel). *J Eur Acad Dermatol Venereol* 2003;17(4):459-60.
27. Chen GY et al. Onychomadesis and onycholysis associated with capecitabine. *Br J Dermatol* 2001;

145:520-1.

28. Maino KL, Norwood C, Stashower ME. Onycholysis with the appearance of a "sunset" secondary to capecitabine. *Cutis* 2003;72:234-6.
29. Munoz A et al. Onycholysis associated with capecitabine in combination with irinotecan in two patients with colorectal cancer. *J Natl Cancer Inst* 2003;16:1252-3.
30. Obermair A et al. Onycholysis of the finger and toenails following the application of high-dose oral etoposide (1250 mg/m^2) given as 200 and 150 mg single doses from days 1-10 every 3 weeks. *Gynecol Oncol* 1995;57:436.
31. Nakamura S et al. Improvement in docetaxel-induced nail changes associated with cyclooxygenase-2 inhibitor treatment. *Clin Exp Dermatol* 2009;34(7): e320-1.
32. Scotté F et al. Multicenter study of a frozen glove to prevent docetaxel-induced onycholysis and cutaneous toxicity of the hand. *J Clin Oncol* 2005;23:4424-9.
33. Heidary N, Naik H, Burgin S. Chemotherapeutic agents and the skin: An update. *J Am Acad Dermatol* 2008;58(4):545-70.
34. Busam KJ et al. Cutaneous side-effects in cancer patients treated with the antiepidermal growth factor receptor antibody C225. *Br J Dermatol* 2001;144(6):1169-76.
35. Chang GC et al. Paronychia and skin hyperpigmentation induced by gefitinib in advanced non-small cell lung cancer. *J Clin Oncol* 2004;22:4646-7.
36. Lacouture ME et al. Analysis of dermatologic events in patients with cancer treated with lapatinib. *Breast Cancer Res Treat* 2009;114(3):485-93.
37. Balagula Y et al. Dermatologic side effects associated with the MEK 1/2 inhibitor, selumetinib. *Invest New Drugs* 2011;29(5):1114-21.
38. Wu PA et al. Prophylaxis and treatment of dermatologic adverse events from epidermal growth factor receptor inhibitors. *Curr Opin Oncol* 2011;23(4):343-51.
39. Schad K et al. Mitogen-activated protein/extracellular signal-regulated kinase kinase inhibition results in biphasic alteration of epidermal homeostasis with keratinocytic apoptosis and pigmentation disorders. *Clin Cancer Res* 2010;16:1058-64.
40. Piraccini BM, Iorizzo M, Tosti A. Drug-induced nail abnormalities. *Am J Clin Dermatol* 2003;4(1): 31-37.
41. Deslandres M et al. Cutaneous side effects associated with epidermal growth factor receptor and tyrosine kinase inhibitors. *Ann Dermatol Venereol* 2008;1:16-24.
42. Galimont-Collen AF et al. Classification and management of skin, hair, nail and mucosal side-effects of epidermal growth factor receptor (EGFR) inhibitors. *Eur J Cancer* 2007;43(5):845-51.
43. Capriotti K et al. Chemotherapy-associated paronychia treated with 2% povidone-iodine: A series of cases. *Cancer Manag Res* 2017;9:225.
44. Hachisuka J et al. Effect of adapalene on cetuximab-induced painful periungual inflammation. *J Am Acad Dermatol* 2011;64(2): e20-1.
45. Lacouture ME, Boerner SA, Lorusso PM. Non-rash skin toxicities associated with novel targeted therapies. *Clin Lung Cancer* 2006; Suppl 1: S36-42.
46. Robert C et al. Cutaneous side-effects of kinase inhibitors and blocking antibodies. *Lancet Oncol* 2005;6:491-500.
47. Fox LP. Nail toxicity associated with epidermal growth factor receptor inhibitor therapy. *J Am Acad Dermatol* 2007;56:460-5.
48. Kiyohara Y, Yamazaki N, Kishi A. Erlotinib-related skin toxicities: Treatment strategies in patients with metastatic non-small cell lung cancer. *J Am Acad Dermatol* 2013;60:463-72.

49. Vogelzang NJ et al. Raynaud's phenomenon: A common toxicity after combination chemotherapy for testicular cancer. *Ann Intern Med* 1981;95:288-92.
50. Sibaud V et al. Dermatological adverse events with taxane chemotherapy. *Eur J Dermatol* 2016;26(5):427-43.
51. Freiman A, Bouganim N, O'Brien EA. Mitozantrone-induced onycholysis associated with subungual abscesses, paronychia, and pyogenic granuloma. *J Drugs Dermatol* 2005;4:490-1.
52. Roé E et al. Description and management of cutaneous side effects during cetuximab or erlotinib treatments: A prospective study of 30 patients. *J Am Acad Dermatol* 2006;55(3):429-37.
53. Robert C et al. Subungual splinter hemorrhages: A clinical window to inhibition of vascular endothelial growth factor receptors? *Ann Intern Med* 2005;143(4):313-4.

第十章

新生物反应

彼得·阿恩·格贝尔(Peter Arne Gerber)

缪 盈 译

一 背景

肿瘤治疗的主要策略包括手术、放疗、药物疗法或其组合。这似乎是一个悖论,特别是放疗和某些抗癌药物可能诱发肿瘤本身的发展。直到肿瘤反应发展的潜伏期可能很短,并且反应可能与病因治疗直接相关甚至在病因治疗下发生。然而,新生物反应也可能在癌症治愈数年后发展,并在长期癌症幸存者出现问题。值得注意的是,在所有器官系统中,这些后续新生物(subsequent neoplasm, SN)被认为是最严重的并发症之一,继发恶性新生物(subsequent malignant neoplasm, SMN)与长期癌症幸存者的死亡率关联性最强[1,2]。

关于皮肤的肿瘤反应,长期癌症幸存者继发的恶性和原位肿瘤几乎完全与放疗相关[3]。然而,传统的细胞毒性化学疗法,特别是选择性的靶向癌症药物,可能引起广泛的良性和恶性肿瘤反应。一方面,简化的传统化疗非选择性地靶向所有快速增殖的身体细胞和组织,这包括癌细胞,也包括造血系统、黏膜或毛囊的健康细胞。因此,不良反应范围从贫血和脱发到黏膜糜烂、呕吐等(图 10-1)。关于肿瘤性皮肤反应,传统化疗与发疹性黑素细

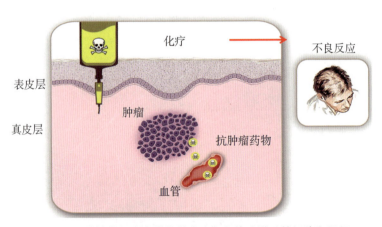

图 10-1 传统的细胞毒性化学疗法靶向快速增殖的细胞和组织

例如癌组织。由于这种作用相对没有选择性,因此会影响具有高增殖率的生理组织,例如毛囊或黏膜。其后果是典型的化疗相关不良反应,例如脱发。图片由 Peter Arne Gerber 和 Holger Schrumpf 设计。

胞斑/痣[4,5]、光化性角化病的炎症[6,7]和化脓性肉芽肿[8]有关。

另一方面，靶向药物在过去 10 年中彻底改变了现代肿瘤的治疗。分子生物学和医学的快速发展推动了它们的发展。事实上，肿瘤特异性细胞和分子特征的识别为设计针对这些靶标的药物提供了机会。理想的情况是，这些靶向药物将优于传统化疗药物，因为它们具有更高的肿瘤定向功效和更低的非定向细胞毒性和不良反应。然而，靶向治疗也可能伴随广泛的特征性毒性。这些与传统化疗的不良反应不同，通常耐受性更好。然而，也可能发生相当严重和令人厌烦的毒性。由于许多已确定的肿瘤靶标也存在于皮肤中，因此皮肤毒性代表了靶向抗癌药物最常见的一些不良反应[9-11]。靶向治疗的肿瘤性皮肤反应包括化脓性肉芽肿[12]、鳞状细胞增生性病变（squamoproliferative lesions，SCPL）和非黑色素瘤皮肤癌（nonmelanoma skin cancer，NMSC）[13-17]，以及发疹性黑素细胞斑/痣[10,18,19]。

二 非黑色素瘤皮肤癌和鳞状细胞增生性病变

在接受 BRAF 靶向治疗的癌症患者中，一种特别重要的 NMSC 是角化棘皮瘤（keratoacanthoma，KA）。KA 发展为孤立的，有时是多发的、外生的、圆顶形肿瘤，具有中央溃疡（图 10-2），其特征是在几周内快速生长。肿瘤被认为是低级别的，在挤压掉中心块碎片后无须治疗即可治愈。光化性皮肤损伤区域出现多个 NMSC 是临床常见的，又称"光化性区域癌变"（图 10-3）[20]。在儿童癌症幸存者中，放疗史与 90% 受影响患儿的 NMSC 发展相关，主要是日光性角化症（actinic keratosis，AK）和鳞状细胞癌（squamous cell carcinomas，SCC）[3]。然而令人惊讶的是，尽管传统化疗具有潜在的免疫调节作用，但并未发现其与传统化疗的阳性史相关（另请参阅"癌症幸存者的皮肤新生物反应"部分）[3]。据报道，抗代谢物羟基脲（HU）发生 NMSC 的风险增加，潜伏期为 2～13 年[21]。其中包括阳光暴露区域的多种侵袭性 SCC、鲍恩病（Bowen disease）和 AK。建议停用 HU 以解决或至少改善各种 HU 相关的鳞状细胞不典型增生。提出的作用方式是 HU 在紫外线照射区域诱导 *p53* 引发角质形成细胞突变[21]。传统化疗主要与先前存在的 NMSC 反应有关，例如 5-氟尿嘧啶（5-FU）诱导 AK 的炎症。发病机制概念提出转化的角质形成细胞对 5-FU 诱发的细胞损伤易感性增高，导致随后的炎症反应[6,7]。

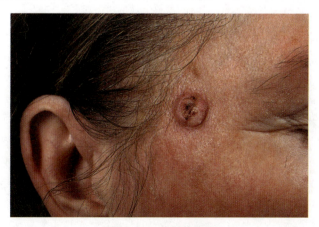

图 10-2　角化棘皮瘤

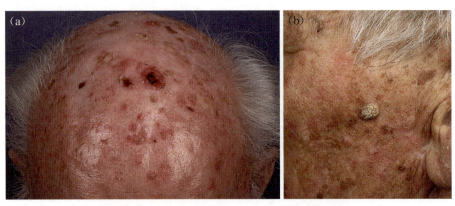

图 10-3 非黑色素瘤皮肤癌(NMSC)的临床表现

(a)头皮的光化区域癌变伴多个日光性角化症;(b)面部和耳部的光化区域癌变伴多种日光性和脂溢性角化症、日光性雀斑样痣和寻常疣。

关于 NMSC 和靶向肿瘤治疗,丝裂原活化蛋白激酶(MAPK;图 10-4)途径的某些激酶抑制剂与 NMSC(AK、SCC、KA)和 NMSC 样所谓的角化性或 SCPL[22]。MAPK 信号转导对实体肿瘤发病机制重要性的一个突出例子是黑色素瘤[23]。激酶 BRAF 的激活突变非常频繁,发生在 40%~60% 的皮肤黑色素瘤患者中(图 10-5)。最近,特定的 BRAF 抑制剂,如维莫非尼或达拉非尼,已被证明可以改善转移性黑色素瘤患者的无进展生存期和总生存期[24,25]。BRAF 抑制剂的应用与一系列特征性皮肤不良反应有关,包括继发性皮肤肿瘤。SCPL 的发展,包括疣状乳头状瘤、脂溢性角化病、寻常疣、KA 和 AK 以及分化良好的皮肤 SCC,可被视为特殊类别,据报道在 10%~30% 的患者中出现(图 10-6)[22,24,26-28]。SCPL 最早可能在 BRAF 抑制剂治疗开始后的 2 周和最长 14 周出现。BRAF 抑制剂诱导 SCPL 的分子分析已检测到高频率的突变 RAS,特别是 HRAS[27,29]。此外,已证明激活的 RAS 会导致 MAPK 信号反常激活和 BRAF 野生型皮肤细胞中的连续肿瘤生长[27]。由于这些皮肤改变显示出与激活 RAS/MAPK 种系突变的一组遗传综合征重叠,例如克斯提洛弹性蛋白缺陷症(Costello syndrome, CS)或努南综合征(Noonan syndrome, NS),因此皮肤不良反应也被称为"RASopathic"[30]。关于 RAF 抑制剂诱导 SCPL 的其他风险因素,在接受维莫非尼治疗患者的 SCPL 中发现了人乳头瘤病毒(HPV)的 DNA。此外,在 HPV 驱动的 SCC 转基因小鼠模型中,维莫非尼治疗可显著增加 SCC 发病率,从 22% 至 70%[31]。

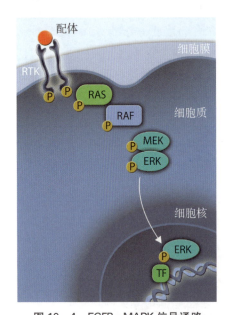

图 10-4 EGFR-MAPK 信号通路

图片由 Peter Arne Gerber 和 Holger Schrumpf 设计。

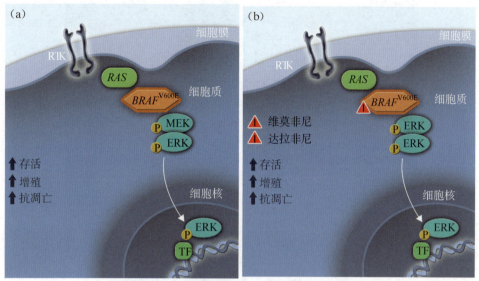
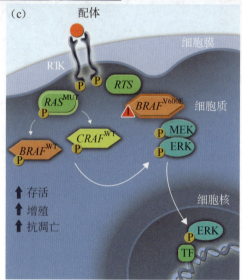

图 10-5　恶性黑色素瘤中的 MAPK 信号转变

(a)激活 *BRAF* 突变(例如 V600E)是黑色素瘤发病机制中的关键点;(b)BRAF 抑制剂(维莫非尼、达拉非尼)显著推进了现代黑色素瘤治疗;(c)RAS 信号的反常激活是 BRAF 抑制剂诱导的鳞状细胞增殖性病变(SCPL)发病机制中的关键点。图片由 Peter Arne Gerber 和 Holger Schrumpf 设计。

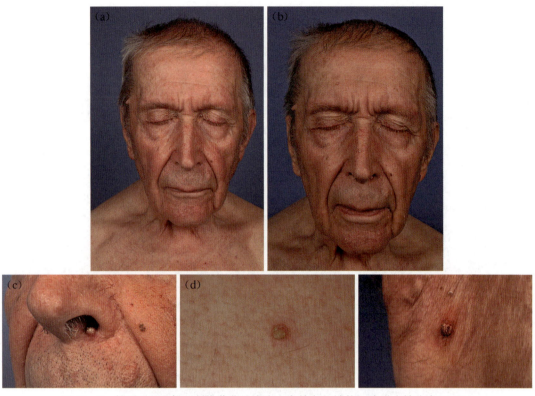

图 10-6 接受 BRAF 抑制剂维莫非尼治疗患者的多处鳞状细胞增生性病变(SCPL)
包括(c)角化棘皮瘤、(d)皮角和(e)疣状乳头状瘤。BRAF 抑制开始后(a)第 3 周和(b~e)第 8 周的患者。

对接受 RAF 抑制剂治疗患者 SCPL 处理和预防的建议包括每 4~6 周定期进行皮肤监测和严格的防晒措施。对于 RAF 抑制剂诱导的肿瘤反应治疗,建议对可疑病变进行全切除手术[32]。然而,出现多处病变的患者也可采用定向破坏性措施进行治疗,例如冷冻疗法,以及用于处理光化区域癌变的被认定的一些疗法,如局部 5-FU、甲醇丁烯醇或光动力疗法(photodynamic therapy,PDT),或其组合,例如病灶强化场治疗(lesion intensified field therapy,LIFT)-PDT[22,33]。最后,口服阿曲汀的成功治疗已被证明[28]。关于阿曲汀的功效,认为维 A 酸可直接与 RAF/MEK/ERK 和 PTEN/PI3K/Akt/mTOR 通路的成分相互作用,并降低 Erk1 活性和 EGF 的分泌[34]。

值得注意的是,由于黑色素瘤治疗的进展,在接受 BRAF 抑制剂治疗的患者中诱导的新生物反应已经变成一个可以忽略不计的问题。事实上,在 BRAF 阳性晚期黑色素瘤患者中,BRAF 抑制剂的单一疗法已被 BRAF 抑制剂(维莫非尼、达拉非尼)和 MEK 抑制剂(曲美替尼、考比替尼)的组合所取代,成为一种新的治疗标准[35]。令人惊讶的是,与各个单一疗法相比,MAPK 通路的两个连贯激酶抑制显著提高了疗效和患者的总体存活率,我们还观察到不良反应的发生率也明显降低[36]。特别是在 BRAF/MEK 抑制剂治疗的患者中,SCPL 的发生率从 BRAF 抑制剂治疗的 10%~30%降至 0%~1%[22,35]。提出的分子机制是在 MEK 水平上反常 RAS 信号转导的抑制。引人注目的是，在"概念验证"观察中，据报道，在 BRAF 抑制剂方案中添加 MEK 抑制剂会导致先前存在的 BRAF 抑制剂诱导的 SCPL 完全消退[37]。

NMSC（包括 SCC）的诱导也与靶向 RAF 的多激酶抑制剂（MKI）有关，如索拉非尼。此外，在接受索拉非尼治疗的 10% 患者中观察到先前存在 AK 的炎症反应[13-17,22]。最后，最近的观察报道，在接受针对转化生长因子-β（抗 TGF-β）的单克隆抗体非苏木单抗治疗的患者中诱发 KA 和 SCC。根据 RAF 抑制剂诱导 SCPL 的发现，作者提出 TGF-β 和 MAPK 通路的交互是最可能的致病分子机制[38]。

三 色素性病变

与药物相关的发疹性痣（eruptive nevi associated with medication，ENAM）已被报道与众多药物有关，包括传统化疗和靶向抗肿瘤药物[5]。ENAM 的诊断可以界定为与药物使用相关的，任何年龄人群在手掌或足底出现黑色素细胞痣＞5 个，除青春期或妊娠期外全身黑色素细胞痣＞10 个[3]，或除青春期或妊娠期外在 6 个月期间全身黑色素细胞痣＞10 个[5]。痣在治疗后数周至数月内出现，通常表现为直径 1～3 mm 的浅褐色至深褐色斑疹（图 10-7）。药物引起的痣通常存在于以下分布区之一：掌跖、局限于躯干或弥漫性，手掌和足底更好发[39]。ENAM 可以根据药物类型进一步分成几个亚型，即 Ⅰa"非生物免疫抑制剂"、Ⅰb"生物免疫抑制剂"、Ⅱa"非生物化学治疗剂"、Ⅱb"生物化学治疗剂"和 Ⅲ"直接黑色素细胞刺激剂"[5]。

与 ENAM（Ⅱa 型）相关的传统化疗药物包括卡培他滨[40]、干扰素 α-2b[41]、环磷酰胺、奥曲肽、多柔比星和柔红霉素[4,6]，以及联合化疗[5,42]。非生物药物诱导 ENAM 的发病机制概念主要提出免疫抑制作用和局部生长因子的连续调节，例如干细胞因子（stem cell factor，SCF）和黑色素细胞生长因子[39,43]。

与 ENAM（Ⅱb 型）相关的靶向抗癌药物包括 EGFR 抑制剂（厄洛替尼）[44]、BRAF 抑制剂（维莫非尼、康奈非尼）[45,46]和多激酶抑制剂（MKI；索拉非尼、舒尼替尼、瑞戈非尼）[18,19,47]，以及抗 CD20 抗体（利妥昔单抗）[5]。据报道，对于 BRAF 抑制剂，ENAM 发生在 10% 受治的患者中[45]。值得注意的是，在接受 BRAF 抑制剂治疗的患者中，有 20% 的患者出现第 2 原发性黑色素瘤（second primary melanomas，SPM）[48]。根据 BRAF 抑制剂和 MKI 诱导 SCPL 和 NMSC 的致病概念，靶向药物诱导 ENAM 和 SPM 是 RAS-RAF-MEK 信号通路的反常活化。同样，概念验证观察报道在升级到 BRAF/MEK 抑制剂组合方案后，BRAF 抑制剂诱导的 ENAM 快速和完全消退[45]。

对接受 BRAF 抑制剂单药治疗的患者预防和管理 ENAM 和 SPM 的建议包括在治疗开始前记录预先存在的黑色素细胞痣（"身体映像"），每 4～8 周进行一次监测访问，包括皮肤镜检查和数字跟踪（如果有），以及采取严格的防晒措施[22]。

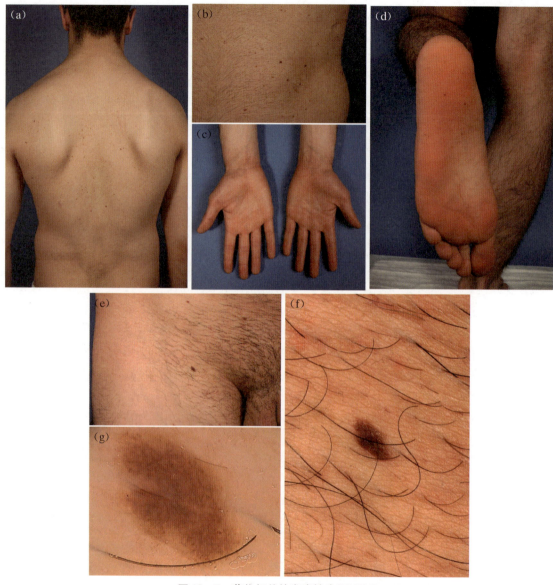

图 10-7 药物相关的发疹性痣(ENAM)

(a~d)背部、腹部、手掌、足底;(e~g)黑色素细胞痣,示大体、细节和皮肤镜图像。

四 化脓性肉芽肿

化脓性肉芽肿(图 10-8)与 5-FU、卡培他滨、甲氨蝶呤和多柔比星等传统化疗以及针对 EGFR(图 10-9)、BRAF 和 CD20 的靶向治疗有关[12,49-52]。肿瘤经常出现在甲周部位。尽管这些临床观察将化脓性肉芽肿的诱导与 EGFR/MAPK 通路的抑制联系起来,但最近的研究已确定激活 *RAF* 和 *RAS* 突变是化脓性肉芽肿发病机制的主要驱动因素[53]。这些看似有争议的发现说明了不同信号通路和激酶在靶向药物发病机制中复杂的相互作用。与在 EGFR/MAPK 靶向药物下其他肿瘤形成的发病模型一致，在 EGFR 和 BRAF 抑制下化脓性肉芽肿的发展导致 MAPK 通路的反常活化[52,54]。然而，化脓性肉芽肿似乎可能只是轻微创伤的结果，并且在接受抗癌药物治疗的患者中，指甲和甲周区域的额外毒性频率增加。

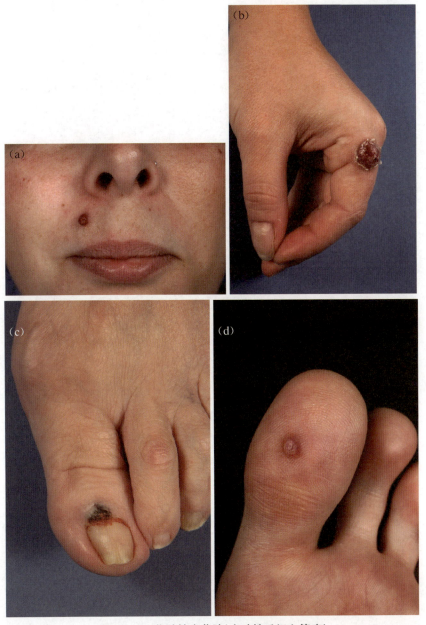

图 10-8 化脓性肉芽肿(小叶性毛细血管瘤)

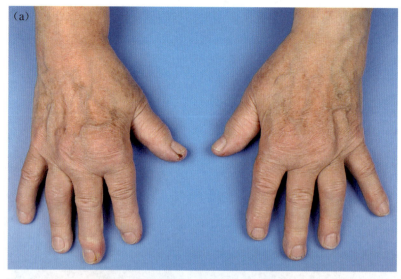

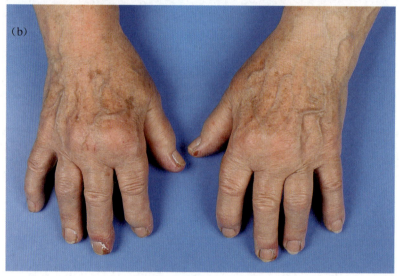

图10-9 接受抗EGFR抗体帕尼单抗治疗患者的皮肤和指甲毒性:化脓性肉芽肿、甲沟炎和裂隙

照片摄于抗EGFR治疗开始后(a)第6周和(b)第8周。

在接受药物抗癌治疗的患者中预防甲周病变和指甲毒性的策略包括避免创伤或对指甲和甲周组织的操作以及随后的皮肤保湿护理[12,50,55]。尤其应避免或谨慎进行美甲、修脚、咬指甲、去除甲小皮等。其他建议包括使用防护手套、棉袜和宽松的鞋子;修剪指甲规则——笔直、避免太短和保持指甲平滑;必要时拜访足科医生;避免使用有毒涂剂和清洁剂[50]。

化脓性肉芽肿的治疗建议主要包括损毁性措施,例如应用液氮进行冷冻治疗,以及局部应用10%硝酸银水溶液、88%苯酚或35%三氯乙酸(trichloroacetic acid,TCA)。此外,可以局部外用或病灶内注射强效糖皮质激素。文献报道的其他病灶内治疗选择是注射乙醇胺、十四烷基硫酸钠或聚多卡醇[49]。然而,这些措施与周围组织坏死的风险相关,因此,为了完整起见,仅在此处列出。更具侵入性的选择包括通过手术刮除、电干燥或切除,以及使用剥脱性 CO_2 或非剥脱性脉冲染料激光(pulsed dye laser,PDL)进行治疗[50]。在严重的情况下,可能需要调整剂量,必要时甚至停止和更换病因性抗肿瘤药物[50]。

五 癌症幸存者的皮肤新生物反应

NMSC 是长期癌症幸存者中最常见的后续新生物,占所有已确认新生物的 40% 以上[1,3]。此外,发生 NMSC 的癌症幸存者在第 1 个 NMSC 后 10 年内发生第 2 个 NMSC 的风险很高[1]。令人惊讶的是,虽然 NMSC 的发展与 90% 的放疗史相关,而这些 NMSC 中有 90% 发生在放疗领域,但没有发现与阳性化疗史有显著关联[3]。据报道,在蒽环类药物暴露方面,NMSC 的风险甚至略有降低[3]。在成年人中,抗代谢物羟基脲与多发性 NMSC 的发生有关。建议停用羟基脲以减少相关肿瘤的发生[21]。

除了 NMSC,癌症幸存者患黑色素瘤的风险更高[56,57]。关于风险因素,仅发现化疗(烷化剂和抗有丝分裂药物)与放疗相结合会增加 SMN 发展为黑色素瘤的风险[56]。儿童时期的化疗是众所周知的过度良性痣发展的危险因素[58]。最后,最近发现嘌呤类似物氟达拉滨可显著增加慢性淋巴细胞白血病/小淋巴细胞淋巴瘤(CLL/SLL)幸存者的黑色素瘤风险,但不会增加其他非霍奇金淋巴瘤(non-Hodgkin lymphoma,NHL)亚型[59]。

六 结语

新生物反应,包括良性和恶性肿瘤,可以由不同的传统化学治疗剂以及靶向抗肿瘤药物诱发。肿瘤科医生应了解各类新生物的潜在谱系和临床表现,以及推荐的处理方案。考虑到靶向治疗领域的动态发展以及针对越来越多不同靶点的新批准药物的数量不断增加,相关新生物反应的范围也将会增加。尽管跟上该领域的这些进展具有挑战性,但这些新的反应也提供了一个机会,可以提高我们对一般皮肤生物学,特别是对上皮肿瘤发病机制的认识。

参 考 文 献

1. Armstrong GT et al. Occurrence of multiple subsequent neoplasms in long-term survivors of childhood cancer: A report from the childhood cancer survivor study. *J Clin Oncol* 2011;29(22):3056-64.
2. Armstrong GT et al. Late mortality among 5-year survivors of childhood cancer: A summary from the Childhood Cancer Survivor Study. *J Clin Oncol* 2009;27(14):2328-38.
3. Perkins JL et al. Nonmelanoma skin cancer in survivors of childhood and adolescent cancer: A report from the childhood cancer survivor study. *J Clin Oncol* 2005;23(16):3733-41.
4. Lotem M et al. Skin toxic effects of polyethylene glycol-coated liposomal doxorubicin. *Arch Dermatol* 2000;136(12):1475-80.
5. Perry BM, Nguyen A, Desmond BL, Blattner CM, Thomas RS, Young RJ. Eruptive nevi associated

with medications (ENAMs). *J Am Acad Dermatol* 2016;75(5):1045-52.
6. Reyes-Habito CM, Roh EK. Cutaneous reactions to chemotherapeutic drugs and targeted therapies for cancer: Part I. Conventional chemotherapeutic drugs. *J Am Acad Dermatol* 2014;71(2):203. e1 - 203. e12; quiz 215 - 16.
7. Krathen M, Treat J, James WD. Capecitabine induced inflammation of actinic keratoses. *Dermatol Online J* 2007;13(4):13.
8. Piguet V, Borradori L. Pyogenic granuloma-like lesions during capecitabine therapy. *Br J Dermatol* 2002;147(6):1270 - 2.
9. Agha R, Kinahan K, Bennett CL, Lacouture ME. Dermatologic challenges in cancer patients and survivors. *Oncology* 2007;21(12):1462 - 72; discussion 1473,1476,1481 passim.
10. Macdonald JB, Macdonald B, Golitz LE, LoRusso P, Sekulic A. Cutaneous adverse effects of targeted therapies: Part I: Inhibitors of the cellular membrane. *J Am Acad Dermatol* 2015;72(2): 203 - 18; quiz 219 - 20.
11. Macdonald JB, Macdonald B, Golitz LE, LoRusso P, Sekulic A. Cutaneous adverse effects of targeted therapies: Part II: Inhibitors of intracellular molecular signaling pathways. *J Am Acad Dermatol* 2015;72(2):221 - 36; quiz 237 - 38.
12. Below J, Homey B, Gerber PA. [Cutaneous side effects of targeted cancer drugs]. *Hautarzt*. 2017; 68(1):12 - 18.
13. Arnault JP et al. Keratoacanthomas and squamous cell carcinomas in patients receiving sorafenib. *J Clin Oncol* 2009;27(23): e59 - 61.
14. Dubauskas Z, Kunishige J, Prieto VG, Jonasch E, Hwu P, Tannir NM. Cutaneous squamous cell carcinoma and inflammation of actinic keratoses associated with sorafenib. *Clin Genitourin Cancer* 2009;7(1):20 - 23.
15. Kong HH, Cowen EW, Azad NS, Dahut W, Gutierrez M, Turner ML. Keratoacanthomas associated with sorafenib therapy. *J Am Acad Dermatol* 2007;56(1):171 - 2.
16. Lynch MC, Straub R, Adams DR. Eruptive squamous cell carcinomas with keratoacanthoma-like features in a patient treated with sorafenib. *J Drugs Dermatol* 2011;10(3):308 - 10.
17. Smith KJ, Haley H, Hamza S, Skelton HG. Eruptive keratoacanthoma-type squamous cell carcinomas in patients taking sorafenib for the treatment of solid tumors. *Dermatol Surg* 2009;35(11):1766 - 70.
18. Jimenez-Gallo D, Albarran-Planelles C, Linares-Barrios M, Martinez-Rodriguez A, Baez-Perea JM. Eruptive melanocytic nevi in a patient undergoing treatment with sunitinib. *JAMA Dermatol* 2013;149 (5):624 - 6.
19. Kong HH, Sibaud V, Chanco Turner ML, Fojo T, Hornyak TJ, Chevreau C. Sorafenib-induced eruptive melanocytic lesions. *Arch Dermatol* 2008;144(6):820 - 2.
20. Stockfleth E. The paradigm shift in treating actinic keratosis: A comprehensive strategy. *J Drugs Dermatol* 2012;11(12):1462 - 7.
21. Sanchez-Palacios C, Guitart J. Hydroxyurea-associated squamous dysplasia. *J Am Acad Dermatol* 2004;51(2):293 - 300.
22. Reyes-Habito CM, Roh EK. Cutaneous reactions to chemotherapeutic drugs and targeted therapy for cancer: Part II. Targeted therapy. *J Am Acad Dermatol* 2014;71(2):217. e1 - 217. e11; quiz 227 - 28.
23. Curtin JA et al. Distinct sets of genetic alterations in melanoma. *N Engl J Med* 2005;353(20): 2135 - 47.
24. Chapman PB et al. Improved survival with vemurafenib in melanoma with BRAF V600E mutation. *N Engl J Med* 2011;364(26):2507 - 16.

25. Hauschild A et al. Dabrafenib in BRAF-mutated metastatic melanoma: A multicentre, open-label, phase 3 randomised controlled trial. *Lancet* 2012;380(9839):358-65.
26. Boussemart L et al. Prospective study of cutaneous side-effects associated with the BRAF inhibitor vemurafenib: A study of 42 patients. *Ann Oncol* 2013;24(6):1691-7.
27. Su F et al. RAS mutations in cutaneous squamous-cell carcinomas in patients treated with BRAF inhibitors. *N Engl J Med* 2012;366(3):207-15.
28. Sinha R, Larkin J, Gore M, Fearfield L. Cutaneous toxicities associated with vemurafenib therapy in 107 patients with BRAF V600E mutation-positive metastatic melanoma, including recognition and management of rare presentations. *Br J Dermatol* 2015;173(4):1024-31.
29. Oberholzer PA et al. RAS mutations are associated with the development of cutaneous squamous cell tumors in patients treated with RAF inhibitors. *J Clin Oncol* 2012;30(3):316-21.
30. Rinderknecht JD et al. RASopathic skin eruptions during vemurafenib therapy. *PLoS One* 2013;8(3):e58721.
31. Holderfield M et al. Vemurafenib cooperates with HPV to promote initiation of cutaneous tumors. *Cancer Res* 2014;74(8):2238-45.
32. Schuurmann M, Ponitzsch I, Simon JC, Ziemer M. Don't miss the base — keratoacanthoma-type squamous cell carcinoma with perineural invasion during BRAF inhibitor therapy for melanoma. *J Dtsch Dermatol Ges* 2015;13(12):1279-81.
33. Braun SA, Gerber PA. Lesion intensified field therapy (LIFT): A new concept in the treatment of actinic field cancerization. *J Eur Acad Dermatol Venereol* 2017;31(5):e232-3.
34. Sachse MM, Wagner G. Clearance of BRAF inhibitor-associated keratoacanthomas by systemic retinoids. *Br J Dermatol* 2014;170(2):475-7.
35. Robert C et al. Improved overall survival in melanoma with combined dabrafenib and trametinib. *N Engl J Med* 2015;372(1):30-39.
36. Sanlorenzo M et al. Comparative profile of cutaneous adverse events: BRAF/MEK inhibitor combination therapy versus BRAF monotherapy in melanoma. *J Am Acad Dermatol* 2014;71(6):1102-1109.e1.
37. Furudate S et al. Keratoacanthoma, palmoplantar keratoderma developing in an advanced melanoma patient treated with vemurafenib regressed by blockade of mitogen-activated protein kinase kinase signaling. *J Dermatol* 2017;44(9):e226-7.
38. Lacouture ME et al. Cutaneous keratoacanthomas/squamous cell carcinomas associated with neutralization of transforming growth factor beta by the monoclonal antibody fresolimumab (GC1008). *Cancer Immunol Immunother* 2015;64(4):437-46.
39. Woodhouse J, Maytin EV. Eruptive nevi of the palms and soles. *J Am Acad Dermatol* 2005;52(5 Suppl 1):S96-S100.
40. Bogenrieder T, Weitzel C, Scholmerich J, Landthaler M, Stolz W. Eruptive multiple lentigo-maligna-like lesions in a patient undergoing chemotherapy with an oral 5-fluorouracil prodrug for metastasizing colorectal carcinoma: A lesson for the pathogenesis of malignant melanoma? *Dermatology* 2002;205(2):174-5.
41. Salopek TG, Mahmood MN. Eruptive melanocytic nevi induced by interferon for nodal metastatic melanoma: Case report and review of the literature. *J Cutan Med Surg* 2013;17(6):410-3.
42. Karrer S, Szeimies RM, Stolz W, Landthaler M. [Eruptive melanocytic nevi after chemotherapy]. *Klin Padiatr* 1998;210(1):43-46.
43. Bovenschen HJ et al. Induction of eruptive benign melanocytic naevi by immune suppressive agents, including biologicals. *Br J Dermatol* 2006;154(5):880-4.

44. Santiago F, Goncalo M, Reis JP, Figueiredo A. Adverse cutaneous reactions to epidermal growth factor receptor inhibitors: A study of 14 patients. *An Bras Dermatol* 2011;86(3):483-90.
45. Chen FW, Tseng D, Reddy S, Daud AI, Swetter SM. Involution of eruptive melanocytic nevi on combination BRAF and MEK inhibitor therapy. *JAMA Dermatol* 2014;150(11):1209-12.
46. Cohen PR, Bedikian AY, Kim KB. Appearance of new vemurafenib-associated melanocytic nevi on normal-appearing skin: Case series and a review of changing or new pigmented lesions in patients with metastatic malignant melanoma after initiating treatment with vemurafenib. *J Clin Aesthet Dermatol* 2013;6(5):27-37.
47. Sibaud V, Munsch C, Lamant L. Eruptive nevi and hair depigmentation related to regorafenib. *Eur J Dermatol* 2015;25(1):85-86.
48. Dalle S, Poulalhon N, Thomas L. Vemurafenib in melanoma with BRAF V600E mutation. *N Engl J Med* 2011;365(15):1448-9; author reply 1450.
49. Curr N, Saunders H, Murugasu A, Cooray P, Schwarz M, Gin D. Multiple periungual pyogenic granulomas following systemic 5-fluorouracil. *Australas J Dermatol* 2006;47(2):130-3.
50. Robert C et al. Nail toxicities induced by systemic anticancer treatments. *Lancet Oncol* 2015;16(4):e181-9.
51. Wollina U. Multiple eruptive periungual pyogenic granulomas during anti-CD20 monoclonal antibody therapy for rheumatoid arthritis. *J Dermatol Case Rep* 2010;4(3):44-46.
52. Sammut SJ, Tomson N, Corrie P. Pyogenic granuloma as a cutaneous adverse effect of vemurafenib. *N Engl J Med* 2014;371(13):1265-7.
53. Groesser L, Peterhof E, Evert M, Landthaler M, Berneburg M, Hafner C. BRAF and RAS mutations in sporadic and secondary pyogenic granuloma. *J Invest Dermatol* 2016;136(2):481-6.
54. Gibney GT, Messina JL, Fedorenko IV, Sondak VK, Smalley KS. Paradoxical oncogenesis — The long-term effects of BRAF inhibition in melanoma. *Nat Rev Clin Oncol* 2013;10(7):390-9.
55. Homey B et al. Escalating therapy of cutaneous side effects of EGFR inhibitors: Experience of German reference centers. *J Dtsch Dermatol Ges* 2012;10(8):559-63.
56. Braam KI et al. Malignant melanoma as second malignant neoplasm in long-term childhood cancer survivors: A systematic review. *Pediatr Blood Cancer* 2012;58(5):665-74.
57. Morton LM et al. Second malignancy risks after non-Hodgkin's lymphoma and chronic lymphocytic leukemia: Differences by lymphoma subtype. *J Clin Oncol* 2010;28(33):4935-44.
58. Hughes BR, Cunliffe WJ, Bailey CC. Excess benign melanocytic naevi after chemotherapy for malignancy in childhood. *BMJ* 1989;299(6691):88-91.
59. Lam CJ et al. Risk factors for melanoma among survivors of non-Hodgkin lymphoma. *J Clin Oncol* 2015;33(28):3096-104.

第十一章

过敏和荨麻疹

卡塔尔多·帕特鲁诺(Cataldo Patruno),玛丽亚·费里洛(Maria Ferrillo),
玛丽亚·瓦斯塔雷拉(Maria Vastarella)

王轶伦 译

一 概述和流行病学

任何抗肿瘤药物的使用都可能使患者暴露于过敏反应(hypersensitivity reaction,HR)的风险中;尽管少见,严重的过敏反应也会发生。药物过敏反应(drug hypersensitivity reaction,DHR)的真实发生率尚不明确,因为通常很难证明药物和这种反应之间的相关性;因此缺乏 DHR 的流行病学数据[1]。某些药物(如紫杉醇)极易引起反应,而仅少数抗肿瘤药物还未有引起 DHR 的报道[2]。

大多数过敏反应是即刻发生的(给药后 1 h 内),但也有许多抗肿瘤药物引起的为非即刻过敏型反应(给药 1 h 以后)的情况[3]。

根据 Gell 和 Coombs 对过敏反应的分类(表 11-1),导致 DHR 的潜在事件是免疫系统对药物的特异性敏感。

表 11-1 Gell 和 Coombs 对过敏反应的分类

类型	免疫反应类型	临床特征
Ⅰ	IgE	荨麻疹,血管性水肿,过敏性休克,支气管哮喘
Ⅱ	IgG 和 FcR	血细胞减少
Ⅲ	IgG 或 IgM 和补体	血清病,Arthus 反应
Ⅳa	Th1	湿疹
Ⅳb	Th2	发疹型药疹,药物超敏反应综合征(DRESS)
Ⅳc	细胞毒性 T 细胞	发疹型药疹,史-约综合征(SJS),中毒性表皮坏死松解症(TEN)
Ⅳd	T 细胞	急性泛发性发疹性脓疱病(AGEP)

然而,由药物不耐受(特异质或假性变态反应)引发的非免疫机制也可能导致反应。药物诱导的假性变态反应或类过敏反应可直接释放组胺,引起面部潮红、皮疹、瘙痒、荨麻疹、

低血压和黏液分泌,这些症状有时很难与真正的 DHR 相鉴别。过敏反应的症状通常比过敏样反应更严重,前者更易发生心血管问题和支气管痉挛,后者更易出现皮肤表现[4]。

在传统的抗肿瘤药物中,铂类和紫杉烷类药物是导致化疗相关过敏反应的主要药物。此外,在过去 10 年中,作为新的肿瘤治疗原则,许多新的生物免疫调节剂进入市场。它们由蛋白质组成,比如细胞因子、单克隆抗体和融合蛋白(可溶性受体)。也有报道这些药物可引起过敏反应,特别是曲妥珠单抗、帕尼单抗、利妥昔单抗和西妥昔单抗。

发生 DHR 的危险因素包括患者和药物相关因素。患者相关因素有年龄、性别(女性>男性)、基因多态性(HLA、药物代谢酶)、病毒感染(HIV、疱疹病毒感染)和交叉反应(化学相关药物过敏反应或化学相关物质的过敏性接触性皮炎史),药物相关因素包括分子大小(高分子物质或高结合力的半抗原)、用法和剂量(表 11-2)。

表 11-2 DHR 的危险因素

患者相关因素	药物相关因素
年龄	分子大小
性别	用法
基因多态性	剂量
病毒感染	—
交叉反应	—

二 诊断

DHR 的诊断基于病史,以及在体和体外试验[2]。

在即刻 DHR 中,皮肤点刺试验是标准试验。如果点刺试验呈阴性,则接着进行皮内试验。虽然皮肤试验是检测高敏感性最简便的方法,但其对化疗药物过敏反应的预测价值尚需要进一步的研究来评估[5]。

大多数药物作为半抗原,无法检测血清 IgE,尤其是目前还没有抗肿瘤药物的商业化 IgE 检测。但一些研究表明,它们可能用于诊断铂类药物引起的过敏反应[6]。当皮肤试验和 IgE 检测不能确定或缺乏时,在体外试验中使用嗜碱性粒细胞活化试验(basophil activation test,BAT)。BAT 通过流式细胞术评估受相关过敏原刺激后嗜碱性粒细胞活化相关蛋白(CD63 和 CD203c 等)的表达[7]。

对于非即刻型 DHR,斑贴试验是主要的诊断性试验。该试验有一些风险和禁忌证,例如有危及生命的过敏反应史。此外,可以使用淋巴细胞转化试验(LTT),这是一种测试记忆 T 细胞反应的体外试验,但须在正确的时间内进行[8]。

在即刻型和非即刻型过敏反应中,药物激发试验是识别 DHR 的金标准,尤其当体外试验结果是阴性的、得不到的或不能确认的时候,必须考虑到体外试验的低灵敏度[9]。药物激发试验应用于一些非常有限的情况下,特别是临床证据表明该种药物有过敏反应,但因没有结构不同却同样有效的其他药物情况下,仍有必要使用该药物,而且使用该药的获益大于风险时。

三、临床特征

DHR 的临床表现取决于所涉及的药物和机制。即刻型 DHR 包括荨麻疹(图 11-1)、血管性水肿、支气管痉挛、呼吸困难、胸腹痛和过敏反应,这些通常是 IgE 介导的反应,而且发生在药物输注期间(表 11-3)。而非即刻型 DHR 的临床表现是多种形态的,如斑丘疹和血管炎(表 11-4)[10]。

表 11-3 抗肿瘤药物即刻型过敏反应的临床特征

即刻型反应	发作时间
过敏反应	给药后 1 h 内
荨麻疹,血管性水肿	
哮喘发作	

表 11-4 抗肿瘤药物非即刻型过敏反应的临床特征

非即刻型反应	发作时间
DRESS、TEN、SJS	给药 2～6 周以后
AGEP	给药 3～5 天以后
湿疹、肝炎、肾炎、光敏	不定

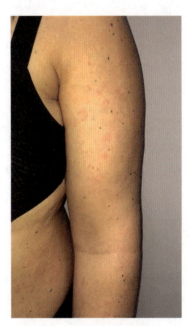

图 11-1 卡铂治疗期间的急性荨麻疹

即刻型 DHR 可分为轻度、中度和重度,并根据 Brown 即刻型过敏反应分级系统进行分类,轻度(1级)反应仅损害皮肤和皮下组织,而中度(2级)和重度(3级)反应可影响心血管、呼吸和神经系统(表 11-5)。

表 11-5 Brown 即刻型过敏反应分级系统

等级	严重度	描述
1	轻度	症状局限于皮肤(如面部潮红)或影响单个器官/系统,症状轻微
2	中度	症状至少涉及两个器官/系统(如面部潮红和呼吸困难),症状轻微,但血压或血氧饱和度没有明显下降
3	重度	症状至少涉及两个器官/系统(如面部潮红和呼吸困难),而且血压和/或血氧饱和度显著下降

(一)铂盐

铂盐(奥沙利铂和卡铂)可引起过敏反应,发生率>5%,多为即刻型 DHR。DHR 通常在多次输注(平均7次)后出现,因为需要反复接触药物才能诱发过敏反应。文献中关于不良反应发生率的估测数据存在相互矛盾[5]。

奥沙利铂与0.5%~25%的轻至中度过敏反应相关,但也与危及生命的1%不良事件相关。在大多数情况下,过敏反应发生在输注末或结束后不久,使用静脉抗组胺剂和糖皮质激素治疗可改善症状。用药前干预在预防奥沙利铂反应方面并不完全可靠,应考虑脱敏方案[6]。

卡铂引起的过敏反应中,大约50%发生在接近用药结束,提示该药需要很长一段时间消退,大约平均在5个化疗周期后出现,而且其对抗组胺药或糖皮质激素反应差[4]。过敏反应是一种潜在的致死性不良事件,常需要终止使用药物。这种反应的风险应与既往药物过敏史、长时间无铂间隔期或大剂量卡铂相关。皮内注射卡铂可用于预测卡铂诱导的严重DHR[7]。

对铂盐诱发过敏反应的诊断,IgE试验的灵敏度低于皮肤试验,但特异度较高。这种测试的一个主要优点是能够在反应发生后不久检测IgE,不需要等待几周才能确定皮肤试验的结果,而这会破坏肿瘤对化疗的反应。另一个优点是能发现交叉反应,在奥沙利铂引起反应的患者中会出现奥沙利铂、卡铂和顺铂的特异性IgE[11]。

(二) 紫杉烷类

紫杉烷类(紫杉醇和多西他赛)是诱发肿瘤患者过敏反应的重要原因。预测因素有3种:年纪轻、过敏史和短时间用药前干预[12]。正如文献报道的,紫杉烷类相关DHR呈剂量和速率依赖。先前的研究表明,紫杉醇和多西他赛引起的过敏反应主要是由药物载体引起的Ⅰ型反应,称为聚氧乙烯蓖麻油,其用于增溶紫杉醇。然而,最近的研究发现,其中一些DHR可能是由IgE介导的。

文献资料报道紫杉醇不良反应发生率高于多西他赛。在意大利的一个病例系列报道中[11],98例过敏反应与紫杉烷类相关(87/240紫杉醇;11/240多西他赛)。紫杉醇(7360次紫杉醇给药中有87次)和多西他赛(912次多西他赛输液中有11次)的发生率均为1.2%。

紫杉烷类药物引起的大部分过敏反应(图11-2)发生在输注开始时,通常发生在第1次或第2次使用药物后[13]。紫杉醇(87%)和多西他赛(100%)引起的过敏反应均出现在治疗开始时[11]。这些反应通常发生得相当快,类似于造影剂引起的DHR。大多数患者在第1次或第2次接触药物后出现反应(仅留下一点点致敏的概率),这似乎很难与IgE介导的机制相协调。这个谜团可以用这样一个事实来解释:对紫杉烷类的敏感性可以在不接触药物的情况下产生,可能是通过空气传播接触。事实上,紫杉醇和多西他赛的前体(巴卡丁Ⅲ和3-脱乙酰巴卡丁Ⅲ)是从不同种类的紫杉树和植物的不同部位包括花粉中分离出来,这可以解释为什么DHR在特应性疾病患者中更为常见[14]。

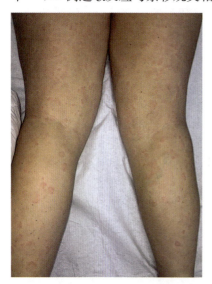

图11-2 首次输注多西他赛后的过敏反应

适当的用药前干预对预防过敏反应极为重要。据报道在没有用药前干预,30%的患者存在 DHR,而使用标准药物用药前干预时,发生率降至 4% 以下。紫杉醇用药前干预方案为口服泼尼松,12 h 前 25 mg,以及氢化可的松(250 mg) + 氯苯那明(10 mg) + 雷尼替丁(50 mg)静脉注射,输注药物前 30 min 给予。多西他赛用药前干预方案包括从化疗前 1 d 开始口服地塞米松 4 mg,持续 3 d,以及治疗当日静脉给予地塞米松 8 mg。

最近有一种新的紫杉醇配方,即白蛋白结合紫杉醇。纳米白蛋白结合紫杉醇(白蛋白结合紫杉醇)不含聚氧乙烯蓖麻油,它使用人血白蛋白将疏水性紫杉醇分子封装在约 130 nm 的颗粒中。与其他紫杉烷类药物相比,白蛋白结合紫杉醇不需要用药前干预来预防 DHR[15]。大多数紫杉烷类药诱导的反应是即刻型的,其体征和症状被认为是嗜碱性粒细胞/肥大细胞脱颗粒的结果。虽然不如即刻型 DHR 常见,但一系列与紫杉烷类药相关的迟发的、可能是免疫介导的过敏反应已被报道。重要的是,迟发性皮肤出疹(最常见的是良性斑丘疹型)可能是下一次输注该药时发生即刻型 DHR 的前奏。SJS 和 TEN 患者中也有报道[17]。

紫杉烷类药皮肤试验可识别由 IgE 介导的敏感患者,是一种有前途的诊断和风险分级工具,可用于对紫杉烷类药有 DHR 患者的处理。应在过敏事件发生后至少 2 周进行皮肤试验,以减少由于 DHR 不应期导致假阴性结果的可能性[17]。

(三) 靶向治疗

单克隆抗体是用于治疗各种人类疾病的创新药物。尽管被设计为比传统化疗更"精准",但靶向治疗经常诱发 DHR。所有单克隆抗体都有过敏反应的报道,特别是曲妥珠单抗、帕尼单抗、利妥昔单抗和西妥昔单抗。

一般来说,DHR 的发生率从西妥昔单抗的 15%~20%(3% 为 3~4 级)和曲妥珠单抗的 40%(<1% 为 3~4 级)到利妥昔单抗的 77%(10% 为 3~4 级)不等[16]。甚至在第 4 次输注后,仍有 30% 的肿瘤患者对利妥昔单抗有过敏反应,而在第 8 次输注后 DHR 的发生率仍有 14%。大约 80% 的致命反应发生在第 1 次输注利妥昔单抗后。

此外,大多数西妥昔单抗的过敏反应发生在首次接触药物后的几分钟内,并且与抗 GA 乳糖-α-1,3-半乳糖的 IgE 抗体相关[17]。半乳糖-a-1,3-半乳糖在西妥昔单抗重链的 Fab 段[18]。对西妥昔单抗的反应似乎是由红肉过敏的相同机制介导的,与肉中的寡糖有关[19]。用药前使用小剂量的倍他米松可以防止大多数患者对西妥昔单抗的过敏反应[20]。

已经报道了对生物制剂的迟发性过敏反应,包括皮疹、血清病样症状、血管炎、多形红斑、SJS 和 TEN。当患者对生物制剂过敏时,快速脱敏是一种开创性的治疗方法,在保护患者免受过敏反应的情况下,将使患者能够接受全剂量的治疗[17]。

(四) 免疫疗法

针对关键免疫检查点的抗体,比如 CTLA-4(伊匹木单抗)和 PD-1(帕博利珠单抗和纳武单抗),已经成为黑色素瘤和其他肿瘤类型(包括非小细胞肺癌和肾细胞癌)的临床有效治疗选择。皮疹、瘙痒和白癜风是最常报道的皮肤不良事件。帕博利珠单抗和纳武单抗的所有级别皮疹的计算发生率分别为 16.7% 和 14.3%。发生时间幅度宽(3 周至 2 年),可能表明对这些药物具有急性和迟发性两类免疫反应,就像许多其他药物引起的皮疹一样。

皮疹通常表现为红斑、丘疹和斑块,主要集中在躯干和四肢,并可能伴有瘙痒。斑丘疹型对外用弱效糖皮质激素有效[21]。

四 处理和结语

众多治疗药物可用于肿瘤的治疗。这些药物在临床疗效方面取得了很大的进步。另一方面,传统治疗和靶向治疗均存在多种不良反应。这些反应可能极大地影响治疗策略。在药物不良反应中,过敏反应仍很常见,而且经常没有得到诊断。中至重度的过敏反应通常需要终止治疗或更换药物,这在很大程度上干扰了对患者的治疗。根据 DHR 的严重程度和治疗方案有几种选择,如明确的停药、用药前措施或脱敏方案。特别是,当患者需要一线治疗时,药物脱敏应被视为标准措施[11]。DHR 后患者的管理涉及风险分级,可以通过快速药物脱敏,或根据初始 DHR 的严重程度和皮肤试验结果进行逐级激惹测试,从而再次启用该药物。

文献中有不同的脱敏方案,但数据存在多样性且有时相互矛盾,这表明尚需要在大量患者中验证脱敏方案,其中包括患有重度 DHR 的患者;理想的还需包括不同人种群体,从而可靠地确定其安全性和有效性。

快速药物脱敏已经被证明是一种有效和安全的方法,可以让数以百计的患者重新应用紫杉烷类药物,包括那些可危及生命的 DHR 患者。非严重迟发性皮肤 DHR 患者可以从快速药物脱敏中受益,因为他们再次接触药物后可能会增加即刻型 DHR 的风险。

这种反应通常持续时间短,在大多数情况下不需要任何特殊治疗,如果不成功,立即使用糖皮质激素就足以控制症状,很少需要重症监护病房干预[11]。

参 考 文 献

1. Demoly P et al. International Consensus on drug allergy. *Allergy* 2014;69:420-37.
2. Raymond B et al. Hypersensitivity reactions from antineoplastic agents. *Cancer Metastasis Rev* 1987;6:413-32.
3. Giavina-Bianchi P et al. Immediate hypersensitivity reaction to chemotherapeutic agents. *J Allergy Clin Immunol* 2017;5:593-9.
4. Brian A et al. Adverse reactions to targeted and non-targeted chemotherapeutic drugs with emphasis on hypersensitivity responses and the invasive metastatic switch. *Cancer Metastasis Rev* 2013;32:723-61.
5. Patil SU et al. A protocol for risk stratification of patients with carboplatin-induced hypersensitivity reactions. *J Allergy Clin Immunol* 2012;129:443-7.
6. Madrigal-Burgaleta R et al. Hypersensitivity and desensitization to antineoplastic agents:Outcomes of 189 procedures with a new short protocol and novel diagnostic tools assessment. *Allergy* 2013;68:853-61.
7. Song WJ et al. Recent applications of basophil activation tests in the diagnosis of drug hypersensitivity. *Asia Pacific Allergy* 2013;3:266-80.

8. Baldo B et al. Adverse reactions to targeted and non-targeted chemotherapeutic drugs with emphasis on hypersensitivity responses and the invasive metastatic switch. *Cancer Metastasis Rev* 2013;32:723-61.
9. Demoly P et al. Determining the negative predictive value of provocation tests with beta-lactams. *Allergy* 2010;65:327-32.
10. Ferrari L et al. Are antineoplastic drug acute hypersensitive reactions a submerged or an emergent problem? Experience of the Medical Day Hospital of the Fondazione IRCCS IstitutoNazionaleTumori. *Tumori* 2014;100:9-14.
11. Castells M et al. Diagnosis and management of anaphylaxis in precision medicine. *J Allergy Clin Immunol* 2017;140:321-33.
12. Aoyama T et al. Is there any predictor for hypersensitivity reactions in gynecologic cancer patients treated with paclitaxel-based therapy? *Cancer Chemother Pharmacol* 2017;80:65-9. Epub 2017 May 10.
13. Markman M et al. Paclitaxel-associated hypersensitivity reactions: Experience of the gynecologic oncology program of the Cleveland Clinic Cancer Center. *J Clin Oncol* 2000;18:102-5.
14. Vanhaelen M et al. Taxanes in *Taxus baccata* pollen: Cardiotoxicity and/or allergenicity? *Planta Med* 2002;68:36-40.
15. Picard M et al. Re-visiting hypersensitivity reactions to Taxanes: A comprehensive review. *Clin Rev Allergy Immunol* 2015;49:177-91.
16. Galvão et al. Hypersensitivity to biological agents-updated diagnosis, management, and treatment. *J Allergy Clin Immunol Pract* 2015;3:175-85; quiz 186.
17. Chung CH et al. Cetuximab-induced anaphylaxis and IgE specific for galactose-alpha-1,3-galactose. *N Engl J Med* 2008;358:1109-17.
18. Munoz-Cano et al. Biological agents: New drugs, old problems. *J Allergy Clin Immunol* 2010;126:394-95.
19. Saleh H et al. Anaphylactic reactions to oligosaccharides in red meat: A syndrome in evolution. *Clin Mol Allergy* 2012;10:5.
20. Ikegawa K et al. Retrospective analysis of premedication, glucocorticosteroids, and H1-antihistamines for preventing infusion reactions associated with cetuximab treatment of patients with head and neck cancer. *J Int Med Res* 2017;45:1378-85.
21. Belum VR et al. Characterization and management of dermatologic adverse events to agents targeting the PD-1 receptor. *Eur J Cancer* 2016;60:12-25.

第十二章

干燥、瘙痒和裂隙

加布里埃拉·法布罗奇尼（Gabriella Fabbrocini），蒂齐亚娜·佩杜托（Tiziana Peduto），
玛丽亚泰雷萨·坎特利（Mariateresa Cantelli）

韩中颖 盛友渔 张 波 译

一 表皮生长因子受体/配体系统与表皮屏障的维持

正常皮肤结构受到表皮生长因子受体（EGFR）抑制剂的显著干扰，基底细胞增殖潜能丧失，角质形成细胞分化受到干扰。由于紧密连接蛋白减少，表皮浅层也受到损害。角质层的形成和功能最终丧失，脱屑增多；体液流失；环境微生物、颗粒物和化学物侵袭增多。这些宿主防御机制的缺陷可能导致微生物的入侵和频繁的皮肤感染。我们反复注意到，缺乏 EGFR 信号的表皮可能导致关键趋化因子和细胞因子的表达和释放紊乱，从而导致免疫细胞群的大量招募和激活，最终表现为皮损[1]。

正如已经充分说明的那样，EGFR 激活和人类皮肤天然免疫机制之间存在协同作用，以最大限度地增强磷酸腺苷（AMP）表达：抑制 EGFR 可阻断中性粒细胞趋化活性和大多数 AMP 的表达。这种缺陷导致皮肤干燥、脱屑和剧烈瘙痒，并导致脱水[2]。

二 EGFR 抑制剂：皮肤-黏膜毒性

EGFR 抑制剂的使用在区域组织层面上出现毒性，其功能严格依赖于 EGFR 和 EGFR 介导的信号转导[3]。

EGFR 抑制剂的主要不良反应是皮肤-黏膜反应，EGFR 在表皮基底层的角质形成细胞、毛囊的外毛根鞘、皮脂腺和小汗腺中表达。在临床上表现为皮疹、丘疹-脓疱、皮肤干燥、毛发生长变化、瘙痒和恶心，较少出现色素沉着、睫毛粗长症、毛细血管扩张和黏膜炎。

皮肤毒性在患者的生活质量中起着关键作用，影响到个体的躯体和心理健康及社会幸福感，并可能导致停药或药物减量。因此，为了在给药、改善患者生活质量和患者预后之间取得平衡，针对皮肤毒性采取适当的治疗是绝对必要的[3]。尤其是使用 EGFR 抑制剂的患者 80% 以上有皮肤干燥症[4]。高龄、特应性体质和既往应用细胞毒性药物是最常见的促发因素。皮肤干燥通常在治疗的第 1 个月和第 2 个月之间出现。到 3 个月时，50% 的患者受到影响；到 6 个月时，接受 EGFR 靶向治疗的患者将 100% 出现一定程度的干燥症[5]。临床可见皮肤干燥、乏脂性皮炎，严重情况下可见皮肤皲裂或裂隙[5]。典型表现为皮肤干燥、脱

屑、瘙痒,通常累及先前痤疮样皮疹分布的相同区域(面部、躯干、四肢末端)(图 12-1)。

皮肤干燥可逐渐演变为真性湿疹,并在继发金黄色葡萄球菌或更罕见的疱疹病毒感染时恶化。有时也可以干痛、结痂的形式出现在手指和足趾的指/趾尖,常伴有指尖、甲襞和指骨间关节的疼痛、裂隙(图 12-2)[6]。

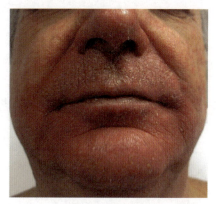

图 12-1　抗 EGFR 治疗患者面部脱屑和干燥皮肤

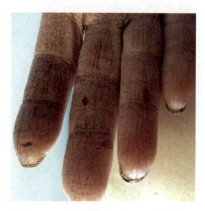

图 12-2　接受抗 EGFR 治疗患者的干燥皮肤和指尖裂隙

皮肤变薄导致皮肤脆性增加,在最严重的区域可见瘀斑[4]。Reguiai 等将干燥症的严重度分为 3 级:1 级,轻微,<10%体表面积,无红斑或瘙痒;2 级,中度,10%~30%体表面积,伴红斑或瘙痒,关键日常活动(烹饪、打电话等)受限;3 级,严重,>30%体表面积,伴红斑或瘙痒,患者的一些特殊关键日常活动(自己洗漱、服药等)受限[7]。

还应考虑到干燥症也可能累及黏膜,尤其是阴道和会阴,排尿时出现不适。皮肤干燥易引起瘙痒,几乎所有患者都会发生。瘙痒通常是全身性的,日间因炎热而加剧,夜间影响睡眠。通常没有原发性皮损;然而,皮肤上可能有许多继发于抓挠的线状抓痕[5]。即使暂停治疗症状也会持续[8]。干燥症的发病机制与 EGFR 抑制剂治疗期间皮肤屏障完整性改变有关。事实上,许多研究表明,EGFR 基因敲除小鼠的皮肤会变得更干燥,表皮颗粒层的兜甲蛋白(loricrin)生成量减少。这种分子在维持表皮屏障功能方面起着关键作用,因为它是角质层中最丰富的蛋白质,除了作为一种重要的屏障蛋白,还有助于防止经皮水分和电解质丢失[4]。

三　皮肤毒性的治疗

(一) 一般预防措施

在开始 EGFR 抑制剂治疗前,每例患者都应接受详细的病史询问,结合客观检查,旨在发现新近或目前的干燥症、寻常痤疮或特应性皮炎。此外,为了降低皮肤毒性的风险,接受抗 EGFR 治疗的患者有必要:

1) 个人护理应使用非侵蚀性洗涤剂,避免使用含酒精的产品(如乳液或香水),这些产品会引起刺激而加剧干燥。

2) 避免穿着化纤类服装,除非使用天然纤维;避免穿太紧的鞋。

3) 使用保湿沐浴露和乳膏(液)保持皮肤水分,缩短沐浴时间。

4) 控制日晒,全年使用高效防晒霜[防晒系数(sun protection factor,SPF)>30],最好使用含有氧化锌或二氧化钛的物理性防晒霜。

(二) 针对各种类型皮肤毒性的治疗策略

EGFR抑制剂治疗过程中出现的不良反应可以通过局部或系统治疗来处理;治疗方法的选择取决于临床类型和严重程度。必须教育和指导患者及时识别和报告任何可能的毒性征象,以便早期干预并确保较好的结果。

为了减轻皮肤干燥,关键要遵循一般预防措施,日常使用润肤霜/乳膏包括衣物遮盖部位,避免过于频繁使用侵蚀性的洗涤剂。与严重瘙痒相关的泛发红斑可能很严重,需外用中效糖皮质激素1~2周(0.05%丙酸倍他米松软膏、氟轻松软膏或0.1%丁酸氢化可的松软膏)。

如果继发抓挠过度,建议局部外用抗生素,如2%夫西地酸软膏、杆菌肽乳膏或2%莫匹罗星乳膏。如果湿疹和脱屑的严重度为3级,建议系统使用糖皮质激素以免发展为严重的剥脱性皮炎(4级毒性)。

干燥症通常伴发瘙痒,可以使用尿素或聚多卡醇(polidocanol)基质润肤剂以及H1抗组胺药(如西替利嗪、氯雷他定、非索非那定和依巴斯汀)进行治疗。

皮肤裂隙可以用封闭性水胶体敷料、修剪指趾甲、使用抗菌溶液(0.025%高锰酸钾)、外用硝酸银溶液以促进愈合。外周皮肤外涂尿素乳膏有利于愈合和预防发病。

参考文献

1. Pastore S, Lulli D, Girolomoni G. Epidermal growth factor receptor signalling in keratinocyte biology: Implications for skin toxicity of tyrosine kinase inhibitors. *Arch Toxicol* 2014;88(6):1189-203.
2. Pastore S, Mascia F, Mariani V, Girolomoni G. The epidermal growth factor receptor system in skin repair and inflammation. *J Invest Dermatol* 2008;128:1365-74.
3. Hu JC et al. Cutaneous side effects of epidermal growth factor receptor inhibitors: Clinical presentation, pathogenesis and management. *J Am Acad Dermatol* 2007;56:317-26.
4. Segaert S, van Cutsem E. Clinical signs, pathophysiology and management of skin toxicity during therapy with epidermal growth factor receptor inhibitors. *Ann Oncol* 2005;16:1425-33.
5. Sinclair R. Anticipating and managing the cutaneous side effects of epidermal growth factor receptor inhibitors. *Asia Pac J Clin Oncol* Mar 2014;10 Suppl 1:11-7.
6. Busam KJ et al. Cutaneous side-effects in patients treated with the antiepidermal growth factor receptor antibody C225. *Br J Dermatol* 2001;144:1169-76.
7. Reguiai Z et al. Management of cutaneous adverse events induced by anti-EGFR (epidermal growth factor receptor): A French interdisciplinary therapeutic algorithm. *Support Care Cancer* 2012;20(7):1395-404.
8. Threadgill DW et al. Targeted disruption of mouse EGF receptor: Effect of genetic background on mutant phenotype. *Science* 1995;269:230-4.

第十三章

放射性皮炎

约翰·戴维·斯特里克利(John David Strickley), 郑彩妍(Jae Yeon Jung)

刘 晓 陶 璐 译

一 术语

戈瑞(gray, Gy)是指每千克物质吸收 1 焦耳的电离辐射能。它是衡量辐射剂量的标准单位。1 Gy = 1 J/kg = 100 rad = 100 cGy。

剂量分割(dose fractionation)是指将总剂量按时间分隔为较小剂量。这种对策可允许用到更高的辐射总剂量,同时最大限度地减少对正常组织的毒性。

增强(boost)是指在常规给药量方案的上限使用额外的辐射来增强对肿瘤的控制。

二 概述

因为放疗对恶性细胞只有适度的特异性,这种治疗对正常细胞总是会引起损害。在放疗强力的细胞毒性作用下,皮肤是最常受伤害部位。>95%的患者在一次性暴露于 8 Gy 的辐射后会出现红斑,这是一种急性放射性皮炎[1]。暴露于 70 Gy 的辐射可导致 50%的患者出现皮肤坏死[2]。

尽管皮肤通常是放疗毒性作用的局外者,但在某些疾病中,皮肤却是靶点。皮肤病的放疗通常用于治疗非黑色素瘤性皮肤癌(图 13-1),但也用于治疗皮肤 T 细胞淋巴瘤、血管肉瘤、梅克尔(Merkel)细胞癌等。一种有效治疗策略的关键要素之一是模式的选择。皮肤科最常用的模式是外照射。其他方式包括近距离放疗、全皮肤电子束(total skin electron beam, TSEB)疗法、调强放疗(IMRT)和立体定向放疗(stereotactic body radiation therapy, SBRT),每一种都有不同的作用,根据病情进展及患者特征选择。

外照射放疗使用光子(X 射线或 γ 射线)或带电粒子(电子或质子)形式的电离辐射。现代外照射采用线性加速器发电产生 X 射线(更简单地称为光子)或电子,前者是皮肤癌治疗中最优选的方式[3]。传统的近距离放疗是通过表面应用器或导管直接应用放射源,而不是电子。新的发展包括使用电子、无放射性核素近距离治疗(如 Xoft®)。TSEB 治疗是将整个皮肤表面暴露于电离电子,并应用于皮肤 T 细胞淋巴瘤。IMRT 的引入是减少对正常组织损伤极其重要的一步。这种图像引导模式使用准直器将辐射束轮廓塑造成恶性肿瘤

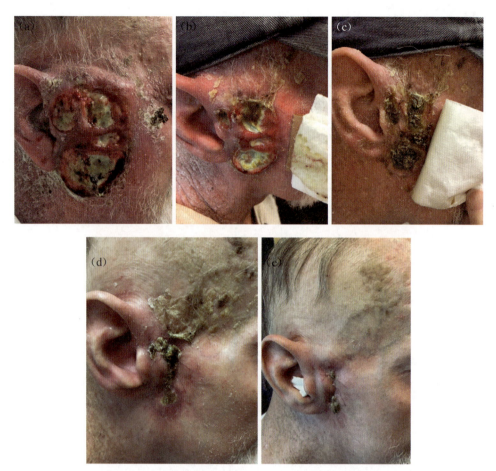

图 13-1　主要接受放疗的无法手术的大鳞状细胞癌患者

出现多种并发症,包括伴有干性和湿性脱屑的急性放射性皮炎。还伴脱发、纤维化和毛细血管扩张的慢性放射性皮炎表现。

的形状,然后从多个角度辐射以分散输送到正常组织的剂量。另一个重大进步是 SBRT,它是一种颅外立体定向放射外科手术,可在射束传输期间补偿目标组织的移动。为此,SBRT 再次利用室内成像来调整患者的呼吸和其他运动,以尽量最小化对正常组织的用量[4]。

剂量分割是提高对恶性细胞相对于正常组织放射敏感性的最重要策略之一。该策略利用肿瘤细胞的某些生物学特性(增殖、细胞周期阶段、修复能力和氧合)来增加对恶性细胞的杀伤并减少对正常组织的损害[4]。分割方案的确定,部分由给定肿瘤的 α/β 比值指导;大多数肿瘤具有较高的 α/β 比值,因此,对较低剂量的更多份额有反应。正如后面所讨论的,这种分割方案是理想的,因为它降低了急性和慢性皮肤毒性的风险。

三　作用机制

电离辐射导致分子发射电子,从而导致高反应性自由基的产生。辐射最重要的细胞靶点是 DNA[4]。辐射与细胞 DNA 的直接相互作用可导致电子丢失,从而导致电离。DNA 和辐射之间的这种直接相互作用被称为"直接辐射作用"。当水的辐射分解后形成自由基(如羟基自由基),然后继续电离 DNA 时,就会发生间接辐射作用[5]。水是细胞中最丰富的分子,相应的,间接辐射作用是造成 DNA 损伤的重要因素。

拥有不成对的电子在尝试建立稳定性中导致分子经历有害的转移突变。这些转移突变导致 DNA 链断裂、核苷酸丢失、核苷酸二聚化等[3]。有丝分裂障碍、细胞凋亡、坏死和衰老都是辐射后细胞死亡的常见模式[6]。在某些情况下,辐射诱导的细胞死亡可导致抗肿瘤免疫反应。这种现象称为远隔效应,可导致未经治疗的转移灶消退,并可被肿瘤免疫调节疗法所增强(如伊匹单抗)[7]。

四 临床表现

(一) 急性放射性皮炎

急性放射性皮炎(图 13-2~图 13-5)是皮肤辐射毒性的最常见表现,在接受放疗的肿瘤患者中发生率>70%[8]。皮肤对辐射的反应因患者因素(如先前存在的状况)和治疗因素(如剂量、部位和分割)而异。病理生理学是多因素的,主要来自辐射引起的炎症、辐射敏感皮肤细胞的直接损伤和伤口愈合中断[9,10]。

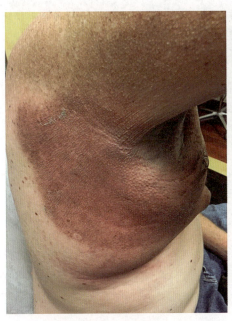

图 13-2 急性放射性皮炎

转移性黑色素瘤患者正在接受腋窝肿瘤的放疗,显示界限分明的红斑和干性脱屑区域,诉轻微瘙痒但无压痛。

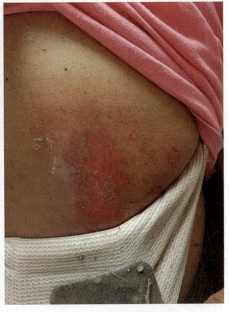

图 13-3 急性放射性皮炎

急性放射性皮炎的转移性肺癌患者,显示表面糜烂(湿性脱屑),诉疼痛和瘙痒。

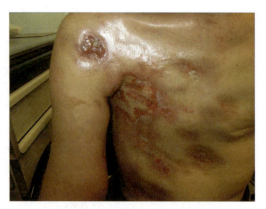

图 13-4　急性放射性皮炎

接受乳房切除术和长期放疗的乳腺癌患者,出现糜烂和潜在的纤维化。

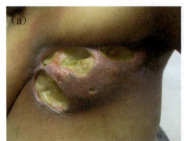 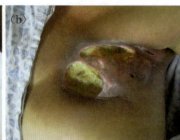 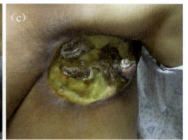

图 13-5　主要接受低剂量放疗 7 个月的乳腺癌患者

(a,b)7月份时;(c)同年10月份时。出现进行性坏死,最终出现干燥的暴露肋骨。

急性放射性皮炎根据临床严重程度的评估进行分级(1~5级);常用的分级系统是不良事件通用术语标准(CTCAE)[11](https://evs.nci.nih.gov/ftp1/CTCAE/CTCAE_4.03_2010-06-14)。1级变化包括轻微的红斑或干性脱屑。1例患有2级放射性皮炎的患者有轻至中度红斑,主要局限于皮肤皱褶处或褶缝的片状湿性脱屑,以及中度水肿。3级显示皮肤褶皱或折痕以外的区域出现湿性脱屑以及轻微擦伤出血。4级预示需要皮肤移植,显示存在坏死或全层溃疡(见图13-5)和自发性出血。最后,5级是死亡。

预防措施包括皮肤护理实践,例如用温和的肥皂清洗和润肤保湿乳液。有证据支持预防性外用糖皮质激素[12]。1级反应的治疗包括润肤保湿剂,因为皮脂腺和小汗腺失去功能;患者应在放疗之间清洁照射区域,这样可以减少细菌负荷。湿性脱屑是2级和3级的特征,表明对感染的易感性增加,因此治疗包括使用水胶体敷料或抗菌银基敷料[13,14];如果怀疑继发感染,应对受影响区域进行皮肤拭子微生物检查。4级反应可能需要清创、皮肤移植和终止放疗。

(二) 继发感染

急性放射性皮炎可出现经久不愈的溃疡、脱屑、大疱、出血和坏死。慢性放射性皮炎也会出现开放性创伤,均会增加感染的风险。继发性感染,或者说继发金黄色葡萄球菌感染

(图 13-6)，由于它可产生超抗原能力，从而加剧辐射毒性的炎症反应[15]；可以像其他皮肤软组织感染一样，采用系统和/或局部抗生素治疗。

(三) 慢性放射性皮炎

慢性放射性皮炎发生于放疗后数月至数年，又称"晚期"反应，可出现在治疗后外观正常的皮肤上。慢性放射性皮炎的发生率与放疗总剂量有关，如给予高剂量（比如 2.5 Gy 或更高）出现的皮肤反应会更严重[16-18]。

常见的晚期表现之一是色素异常（图 13-7），通常是在上皮细胞再生中由炎症后变化所致。色素异常也可以作为一种早期反应出现。同样，坏死也是急性期（见图 13-5）和慢性期（图 13-10）两者的表现。对放射敏感的毛囊和外分泌汗腺受损后可分别继发脱发（见图 13-1e、图 13-8）和闭汗（图 13-9）[19]，并均可见于急性期。皮肤萎缩见于晚期，与辐射诱导的血管损伤和成纤维细胞改变相关[14]。其他可能的慢性或晚期改变将单独介绍，这些表现通常可重叠出现。

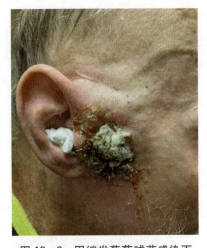

图 13-6 因继发葡萄球菌感染而被忽略的皮肤鳞状细胞癌患者

患处出现恶臭的脓液，伴有疼痛和压痛，周围可见红斑和干性脱屑。

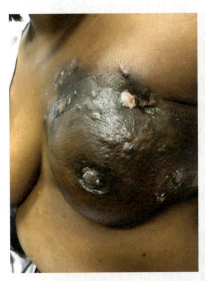

图 13-7 慢性放射性皮炎之色素异常

乳腺癌患者放疗后出现炎症后过度色素沉着，此外出现皮肤水肿（橘皮样外观），并伴乳房沉重和疼痛。

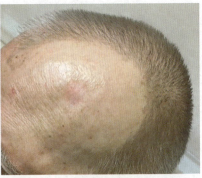

图 13-8 慢性放射性皮炎之脱发

头皮非典型纤维黄色瘤患者放疗后，在治疗区域可见边界明显的斑片状脱发。

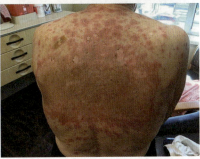

图 13-9 慢性放射性皮炎之狼疮样反应

非小细胞肺癌患者在同步放化疗（顺铂和培美曲塞）后，放射部位出现狼疮样药物反应，可能与皮肤附属器的缺失有关。

(四)辐射诱导的纤维化

受辐射的正常组织(如皮肤、肺和肠道)的纤维化是一种晚期反应,可留下明显的功能和外观方面的后遗症(图 13-10~图 13-12)。放射性纤维化(radiation-induced fibrosis,RIF)主要由细胞因子,尤其是 TGF-β 所介导[20]。辐射还诱导成纤维细胞祖细胞的终末分化,从而产生原纤维性非典型纤维细胞[21]。RIF 的药物治疗旨在阻断炎症通路和自由基损伤,治疗方案包括肌内注射超氧化物歧化酶或己酮可可碱,可单独或与维生素 E 联合使用[22,23],以及物理治疗和按摩[24]。

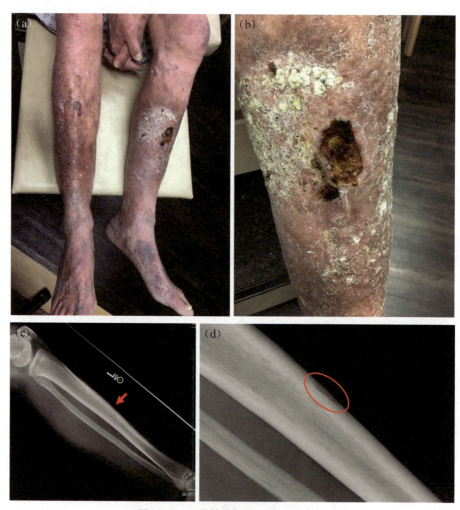

图 13-10 慢性放射性皮炎小腿表现

(a)复发性鳞状细胞癌患者放疗后,多发静脉曲张并愈合不良;(b)放疗 2 年后,左腿进行性纤维化,伴木质样硬结和持续脱屑;(c、d)出现溃疡并导致骨侵蚀,与放射性坏死一致。

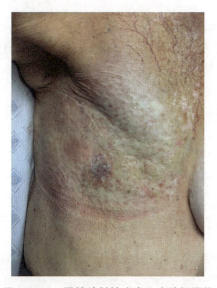

图 13-11 慢性放射性皮炎之皮肤纤维化

乳腺癌患者在乳房切除和放疗后出现皮肤纤维化,束缚并限制了她的活动能力,此外还伴有广泛的毛细血管扩张。

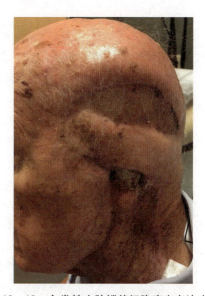

图 13-12 多发性皮肤鳞状细胞癌患者治疗后

该患者在接受局部广泛切除、颈部清创、皮肤移植和放疗后,出现慢性纤维化和颞骨暴露。

(五)毛细血管扩张症

辐射区皮肤出现的毛细血管扩张早已被当作研究慢性放射性皮炎发病率的终点表现[2,18,25]。毛细血管扩张症是真正的晚期表现(图 13-13),它在放疗后数月至数年内出现,之后并不断进展[17],其发病率和潜伏期呈剂量依赖性,较大的辐射量和剂量分割将致发病率升高、潜伏期缩短[17]。暴露量达 65 Gy 后,50% 的患者在 5 年内出现毛细血管扩张症[2]。

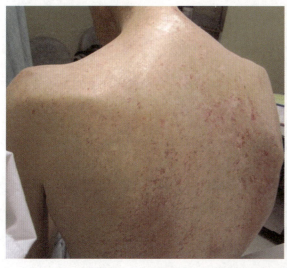 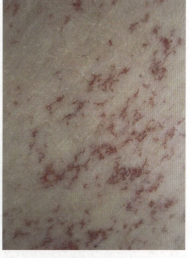

图 13-13 接受造血细胞移植治疗的非霍奇金淋巴瘤患者

该患者全身放疗后出现泛发的毛细血管扩张。

虽然确切的发病机制尚不清楚,推测与电离辐射损伤内皮细胞及产生微血栓有关。也有相互矛盾的数据表明,可能与早期出现的湿性脱屑有关,表明浅表毛细血管丛损伤可能参与发病[25]。已有证据表明脉冲染料激光治疗有效[26]。

(六) 放射记忆反应

放射记忆性皮炎是发生于先前接受过放疗的皮肤部位的一种药物不良反应(图13-14)。典型表现是对化疗药物反应,出现在用药后数天内,并持续至放疗结束后的数月内[27]。放射记忆性皮炎与急性放射性皮炎有许多共同特征,其严重程度不一,可能表现为红斑、水肿、水疱、坏死和溃疡[14],也可见荨麻疹样病变。放射记忆性皮炎的病因尚不清楚,局部外用糖皮质激素的疗效并不明确[27],可通过减量或停止致病药物来控制。

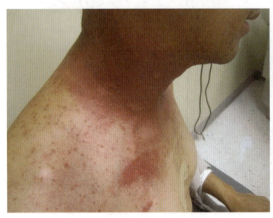

图 13-14 接受放疗的头颈部肿瘤患者

该患者在应用 EGFR 抑制剂后,放射野出现红色斑块。

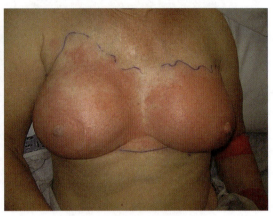

图 13-15 水肿和乳腺炎

接受保留皮肤的乳房切除术及放疗的乳腺癌患者,双侧乳房出现疼痛性红斑和水肿性斑块。

(七) 水肿/乳腺炎

水肿是放疗的急性和慢性反应的主要表现之一。急性水肿可能继发于放射引起的炎症、微血栓和内皮细胞损伤。就乳房而言,接受放疗的乳房体积和提升放疗量等因素可能会增加慢性水肿的风险[28],常见的临床表现包括橘皮样变、乳房沉重、红斑、疼痛、皮肤增厚、色素沉着和凹陷(见图 13-7,图 13-15)[29]。有趣的是,橘皮样变可能引起临床医生对继发恶变(如炎性癌)的怀疑,从而导致不必要的检查。

在接受辅助性放疗的乳腺癌患者中,淋巴水肿的发病率也有所增加[30]。与乳房放疗后出现的水肿不同,前者淋巴水肿更易出现在上肢,这可能与放射性纤维化导致的淋巴管阻塞有关。

(八) 放射后硬斑病

放射后硬斑病(radiation-induced morphea,RIM)是一种罕见的晚期反应,在接受放疗的乳腺癌患者中的发病率约为0.2%，潜伏期为1~12个月[31,32]。与放射诱导的纤维化不同，RIM具有明显的免疫反应成分，即分为两个阶段（图13-16）。第1个阶段是"炎症期"，临床表现为红斑、水肿性斑块；第2个阶段是"燃尽期"，其特征是硬结、紫罗兰变色和疼痛[32]。目前对于该种罕见病症的诊疗尚无共识，建议按斑块状硬斑病的标准疗法处理[32]。

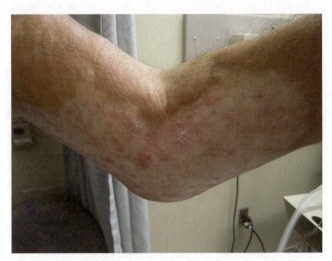

图13-16　皮肤B细胞淋巴瘤和病理性骨折的患者放疗后
患者出现渐进性硬化的斑块，限制了运动范围，皮损区色素减退和毛细血管扩张。

参 考 文 献

1. McLean AS. Early adverse effects of radiation. *Br Med Bull* 1973;29(1):69-73.
2. Emami B et al. Tolerance of normal tissue to therapeutic irradiation. *Int J Radiat Oncol Biol Phys* 1991;21(1):109-22.
3. Gunderson LL, Tepper JE, Bogart JA. *Clinical Radiation Oncology*. Philadelphia, PA: Elsevier; 2016.
4. Abeloff MD. *Abeloff's Clinical Oncology*. Philadelphia, PA: Churchill Livingstone/Elsevier; 2014.
5. Hutchinson F. Molecular basis for action of ionizing radiations. *Science* 1961;134(3478):533-8.
6. Eriksson D, Stigbrand T. Radiation-induced cell death mechanisms. *Tumour Biol* 2010;31(4):363-72.
7. Postow MA et al. Immunologic correlates of the abscopal effect in a patient with melanoma. *N Engl J Med* 2012;366(10):925-31.
8. Hickok JT, Morrow GR, Roscoe JA, Mustian K, Okunieff P. Occurrence, severity, and longitudinal course of twelve common symptoms in 1129 consecutive patients during radiotherapy for cancer. *J Pain Symptom Manage* 2005;30(5):433-42.
9. Boxman I, Lowik C, Aarden L, Ponec M. Modulation of IL-6 production and IL-1 activity by keratinocyte-fibroblast interaction. *J Invest Dermatol* 1993;101(3):316-24.
10. Bernstein EF et al. Healing impairment of open wounds by skin irradiation. *J Dermatol Surg Oncol*

1994;20(11):757-60.

11. National Cancer Institute. Common Terminology Criteria for Adverse Events v4.0. National Insitutes of Health, 2009.
12. Salvo N et al. Prophylaxis and management of acute radiation-induced skin reactions: A systematic review of the literature. *Curr Oncol* 2010;17(4):94-112.
13. Maddocks-Jennings W, Wilkinson JM, Shillington D. Novel approaches to radiotherapy-induced skin reactions: A literature review. *Complement Ther Clin Pract* 2005;11(4):224-31.
14. Hymes SR, Strom EA, Fife C. Radiation dermatitis: Clinical presentation, pathophysiology, and treatment 2006. *J Am Acad Dermatol* 2006;54(1):28-46.
15. Archambeau JO, Pezner R, Wasserman T. Pathophysiology of irradiated skin and breast. *Int J Radiat Oncol Biol Phys* 1995;31(5):1171-85.
16. Turesson I. The progression rate of late radiation effects in normal tissue and its impact on dose-response relationships. *Radiother Oncol* 1989;15(3):217-26.
17. Van Limbergen E, Rijnders A, van der Schueren E, Lerut T, Christiaens R. Cosmetic evaluation of breast conserving treatment for mammary cancer. 2. A quantitative analysis of the influence of radiation dose, fractionation schedules and surgical treatment techniques on cosmetic results. *Radiother Oncol* 1989;16(4):253-67.
18. Johns H, Morris WJ, Joiner MC. Radiation response of murine eccrine sweat glands. *Radiother Oncol* 1995;36(1):56-64.
19. Schultze-Mosgau S et al. Transforming growth factor beta1 and beta2 (TGFbeta2/TGFbeta2) profile changes in previously irradiated free flap beds. *Head Neck* 2002;24(1):33-41.
20. Herskind C et al. Fibroblast differentiation in subcutaneous fibrosis after postmastectomy radiotherapy. *Acta Oncol* 2000;39(3):383-8.
21. Delanian S, Baillet F, Huart J, Lefaix JL, Maulard C, Housset M. Successful treatment of radiation-induced fibrosis using liposomal Cu/Zn superoxide dismutase: Clinical trial. *Radiother Oncol* 1994;32(1):12-20.
22. Delanian S, Balla-Mekias S, Lefaix JL. Striking regression of chronic radiotherapy damage in a clinical trial of combined pentoxifylline and tocopherol. *J Clin Oncol* 1999;17(10):3283-90.
23. Bourgeois JF, Gourgou S, Kramar A, Lagarde JM, Guillot B. A randomized, prospective study using the LPG technique in treating radiation-induced skin fibrosis: Clinical and profilometric analysis. *Skin Res Technol* 2008;14(1):71-6.
24. Bentzen SM, Overgaard M. Relationship between early and late normal-tissue injury after postmastectomy radiotherapy. *Radiother Oncol* 1991;20(3):159-65.
25. Lanigan SW, Joannides T. Pulsed dye laser treatment of telangiectasia after radiotherapy for carcinoma of the breast. *Br J Dermatol* 2003;148(1):77-9.
26. Camidge R, Price A. Characterizing the phenomenon of radiation recall dermatitis. *Radiother Oncol* 2001;59(3):237-45.
27. Hill A, Hanson M, Bogle MA, Duvic M. Severe radiation dermatitis is related to Staphylococcus aureus. *Am J Clin Oncol* 2004;27(4):361-3.
28. Kelemen G, Varga Z, Lazar G, Thurzo L, Kahan Z. Cosmetic outcome 1-5 years after breast conservative surgery, irradiation and systemic therapy. *Pathol Oncol Res* 2012;18(2):421-7.
29. Verbelen H, Gebruers N, Beyers T, De Monie AC, Tjalma W. Breast edema in breast cancer patients following breast-conserving surgery and radiotherapy: A systematic review. *Breast Cancer Res Treat* 2014;147(3):463-71.
30. Kissin MW, della Rovere G Q, Easton D, Westbury G. Risk of lymphoedema following the treatment

of breast cancer. *Br J Surg* 1986;73(7):580-4.
31. Bleasel NR, Stapleton KM, Commens C, Ahern VA. Radiation-induced localized scleroderma in breast cancer patients. *Australas J Dermatol* 1999;40(2):99-102.
32. Spalek M, Jonska-Gmyrek J, Galecki J. Radiation-induced morphea — A literature review. *J Eur Acad Dermatol Venereol* 2015;29(2):197-202.

图书在版编目(CIP)数据

肿瘤治疗的皮肤反应/(意)加布里埃拉·法布罗奇尼(Gabriella Fabbrocini),(美)马里奥·拉库蒂尔(Mario E. Lacouture),(美)安东内拉·托斯蒂(Antonella Tosti)主编;盛友渔,张波主译.—上海:复旦大学出版社,2023.6
(皮肤病治疗系列)
书名原文:Dermatologic Reactions to Cancer Therapies
ISBN 978-7-309-16845-7

Ⅰ.①肿… Ⅱ.①加… ②马… ③安… ④盛… ⑤张… Ⅲ.①肿瘤-治疗-影响-皮肤病 Ⅳ.①R730.5②R751

中国国家版本馆 CIP 数据核字(2023)第 086181 号

Dermatologic Reactions to Cancer Therapies 1st Edition/by Fabbrocini, Gabriella; Lacouture, Mario; Tosti, Antonella/ ISBN: 978 – 1138633254

Copyright © 2019 by Taylor & Francis Group, LLC.

Authorized translation from the English language edition published by CRC Press, a member of the Taylor & Francis Group, LLC. All rights reserved;本书原版由 Taylor & Francis 出版集团旗下,CRC 出版公司出版,并经其授权翻译出版。版权所有,侵权必究。
Chinese Simplified language edition published by FUDAN UNIVERSITY PRESS CO., LTD. Copyright 2023. This edition is authorized for sale throughout Mainland of China. No part of the publication may be reproduced or distributed by any means, or stored in a database or retrieval system, without the prior written permission of the publisher. 本书中文简体翻译版授权由复旦大学出版社有限公司独家出版并限在中国大陆地区销售。未经出版者书面许可,不得以任何方式复制或发行本书的任何部分。
Copies of this book sold without a Taylor & Francis sticker on the cover are unauthorized and illegal. 本书封底贴有 Taylor & Francis 公司防伪标签,无标签者不得销售.
上海市版权局著作权合同登记号 图字 09-2022-0830

肿瘤治疗的皮肤反应

[意]加布里埃拉·法布罗奇尼(Gabriella Fabbrocini)
[美]马里奥·拉库蒂尔(Mario E. Lacouture)   主编
[美]安东内拉·托斯蒂(Antonella Tosti)
盛友渔　张　波　主译
责任编辑/贺　琦

复旦大学出版社有限公司出版发行
上海市国权路 579 号　邮编:200433
网址:fupnet@fudanpress.com　http://www.fudanpress.com
门市零售:86-21-65102580　团体订购:86-21-65104505
出版部电话:86-21-65642845
浙江新华数码印务有限公司

开本 787×1092　1/16　印张 11.25　字数 260 千
2023 年 6 月第 1 版
2023 年 6 月第 1 版第 1 次印刷

ISBN 978-7-309-16845-7/R·2041
定价:150.00 元

如有印装质量问题,请向复旦大学出版社有限公司出版部调换。
版权所有　　侵权必究